Light and Laser Therapy:
CLINICAL PROCEDURES

Sixth Edition

By Curtis Turchin, MA, DC

Disclaimer

It is the responsibility of the practitioner to gain the knowledge of and comply with federal, state and local laws regarding the use of lasers for the treatment of any condition. The content and information in this book is educational only and is designed as an addendum to formal training in laser therapy. It is not a complete course and should not be relied upon for the purpose of treating an individual.

This book is not a substitute for professional medical advice, care, diagnosis or treatment. The treatment of any disease or syndrome should be under the auspices of a qualified physician or therapist.

Dr. Curtis Turchin does not warrant or assume any legal liability or responsibility for the accuracy, completeness, or usefulness of any information, apparatus, product or process disclosed in his book, seminars, or other educational activities. Therefore, Dr. Curtis Turchin is not liable for any kind of loss, risk, or other problem, which is sustained as a result of consulting this book or from using information obtained in any of his books or seminars.

Contact Information

Websites:
www.CurtisTurchin.com
www.GentleMobilization.com

Phone:
Dr. Turchin 707-206-7272

ISBN 978-0-9983910-0-7

Printed in the United States

Introduction: Using This Book

This is a clinical text to help you effectively use light therapy in your clinic. It is designed for almost any type of light therapy product, whether you use a laser or LED, a cluster or a point probe or any other type of therapeutic light device.

Order of Book

The treatment chapters are divided into anatomical regions of the body. The areas are Head and Face, Spine and Pelvis, Upper Extremity, Lower Extremity, Brain, and Systemic conditions. Within each anatomical region, the conditions are in alphabetic order. All diagrams are grouped at the end of each anatomical region so that you can refer to either the text or the diagram, depending on your clinical need.

SOAP Notes

Healthcare demands that practitioners document their findings. For that reason, each condition is organized by the SOAP format. This refers to the Subjective Symptoms, Objective Findings, Assessment, and treatment Plan. This has been designed to help you understand the condition and aid in organizing your assessment and treatment of the patient. There are two "P's." One Plan is your laser treatment Plan and the other is your adjunctive treatment Plan. Because there are a wide variety of modalities available, only the most commonly used adjunctive treatment techniques are included.

Diagrams

In the diagrams, the stationary application of light to a single point on the skin is represented by dots and arrows. The type of small point probe used in auriculotherapy, laser acupuncture, even laser clusters can apply light to a discrete point. For ease of use, the diagrams are only front and back views of the body. Therefore, any point that is applied to the side of the body not pictured is noted by an arrow and the frontal, visible view of the skin is demonstrated by a dot. These points correspond to anatomical locations, not acupuncture points.

Shading denotes that the light is applied in smooth, even strokes called Painting, which is like a slower, more methodical ultrasound application. This is described in the first chapter, Science of Laser Therapy. Most conditions respond to both Point and Painting techniques.

Recommended Dosages

The recommended dosages in this text are based on using a laser with a total output power of between 10 and 10,000 mW. **Please refer to the chart at the beginning of each DIAGRAM section for details on dosages for any laser between 10 and 10,000 mW.**

Ice and Heat

When the application of ice or heat is recommended, it is assumed that the patient can, depending on the practitioner's bias, use ice in the most acute stage, progress to alternating ice and heat as they become subacute, and use heat when the condition is not characterized by serious inflammation.

Suggestions

Light and laser therapy is a new science compared to other modalities used in rehabilitation. Thus, our understanding is changing quickly. If you have information that you feel should be included in this book, or you find something inconsistent with research or your experience, please feel free to email the author. His email address is CurtisTurchin@gmail.com.

TABLE OF CONTENTS

Science of Laser Therapy

Overview of Light and Laser Therapy

This book has been designed as a handbook for the clinical use of laser and LED therapy. Although it includes a short overview of physics, physiology, and the history of laser, these subjects have been purposely limited to maintain the focus on the clinical aspects of laser therapy.

History

The ancient Greeks, Romans, and Egyptians used light therapy and applied heat to tender points in the human body to relieve symptoms of many syndromes.

In 1903, Nils Finsen, a Danish medical doctor, was given the Nobel Prize for successfully treating tuberculosis, rickets and lupus vulgaris with ultraviolet light. This was the first recognized application of artificial light to cure disease.

Later, in 1916, Albert Einstein proposed the basic idea underlying laser operation. The invention of the laser can be dated to 1958 with the publication of the scientific paper, Infrared and Optical Masers, by Arthur L. Schawlow and Charles H. Townes, who worked at Bell Labs. However, it was not until 1960 that Ted Maiman made the first red ruby laser.

In 1923, the Russian researcher Alexander Gurwitsch first detected that cells emit infrared light as a means of intercellular communication. He observed that this light could be transmitted from a test tube to another adjacent one without any physical contact between them. He termed this infrared emission "mitogenetic radiation."

In 1967, Dr. Endre Mester, a professor of surgery in Hungary, performed a revolutionary series of experiments that first documented the healing effect of lasers. In his earliest study he discovered that tissue growth was accelerated with laser therapy. His later experiments documented not only improved healing with light therapy, but also demonstrated that the healing was a systemic and not a local phenomenon. His work stimulated many other researchers in Europe and Eastern Europe to appreciate the value of laser therapy, long before it was appreciated in Asia, Africa, and the Americas.

By the 1970s, laser therapy was beginning to attract attention in Eastern Europe, China, and the Soviet Union; thus, much of the early research emanates from these regions. Over the following ten years, laser therapy spread to Western Europe and quickly became popular as a physical therapy modality. However, many of the lasers used during this period produced only 5 to 50 mW of power and lacked the effectiveness of modern, more powerful lasers.

There has been a recent surge in the use of medical lasers all over the world, particularly in surgery, dentistry, and physical therapy. In the areas of medicine and dentistry, lasers are well known for being extremely precise cutting instruments that lessen the trauma of traditional surgery. In the area of physical therapy, light is being used by physical and occupational therapists, chiropractors, osteopaths, and acupuncturists because of its ability to relieve pain, stimulate healing, and create a wide variety of beneficial systemic effects.

Basic Physics of Laser Radiation

Laser (L.A.S.E.R.) is an acronym for Light Amplification via Stimulated Emission of Radiation. This means that the photons are amplified by the physical processes of the laser design. There are a number of terms that are presently being used to describe Low Level Laser Therapy including: low level laser therapy (LLLT), photomedicine, soft laser, low intensity laser therapy (LILT), cold laser therapy, photonic stimulation, photobiomodulation, light therapy, and many others.

The term Low Level Laser Therapy assumes that the laser emission is low enough so that the treated tissue temperature does not rise more than a few degrees Celsius above normal body temperature. Thus, there is no significant heating effect as there is with higher power lasers.

There are three different parts to a laser: an energy source, a laser material that absorbs this energy and emits it as light, and a cavity that makes this light resonate and channels it into a narrow beam. Within the cavity, very high circulating photon densities stimulate the emission of light from the energized laser material. This design creates a powerful beam of billions of photons, unique to lasers and differentiating them from lower intensity light sources like LEDs.

Lasers Compared to LEDs

In the area of physical therapy two types of light sources are used. They are Laser Diodes (LD) and Light Emitting Diodes (LED). Usually they are visible red (VR) or infrared (IR). Most of the popular diodes emit light in the 600–900 nanometer wavelength range. Lasers are monochromatic, thus emitting a single color of light. To the naked eye, LEDs also emit a single color; however, they actually emit over a narrow wavelength range of about 30 nm.

Lasers are Coherent, LEDs are Non-Coherent

The photons emanating from a laser are highly organized, directional and termed "coherent light". Note in the picture below how the laser light is coherent, or "in-phase" and the LED light is non-coherent or "out of phase."

Notice how the laser light waves are "in-phase"

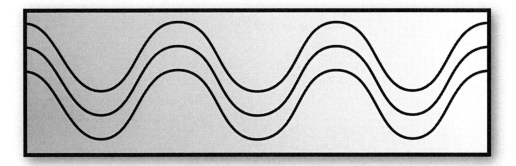

Notice how the LED light waves are "out of phase"

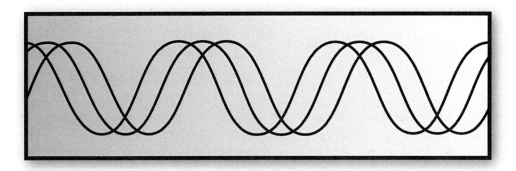

Because laser light is coherent, brighter, and more directional then LEDs, it is recommended for treating conditions in the body when depth of penetration is important, while LEDs are used when more superficial effects are desired.

LEDs are extremely cost effective for many problems. Also, the most powerful LEDs can have effects that are similar to lasers. Thus, higher power LEDs may be as effective as a lower power laser and can provide effective deep treatment when used properly. For example, a 2,000 mW LED at a wavelength of 850 nm could provide more potent and deeper treatment than a 100 mW, 635 nm wavelength laser. The combination of the longer wavelength (which penetrates more deeply) with 20 times the power, makes the LED a more effective modality.

So, it is this coherence and brightness that differentiate lasers from all other light sources. Coherence, by energizing the photons and giving them direction and organization, creates a brighter, more active beam of light. By producing a more powerful, smaller, and narrower beam, it is possible to treat areas of the body both deeply and accurately. A phenomenon called "laser speckling" occurs when the coherent light of a laser contacts almost any surface and produces interference effects that are a unique characteristic of the coherence of a laser.

How Do We Measure Wavelength?

Light travels in a wave as depicted in the diagram below. We can characterize the light by its wavelength, which is the distance between successive peaks (or valleys) in the wave. We measure the wavelength of light in nanometers (nm).

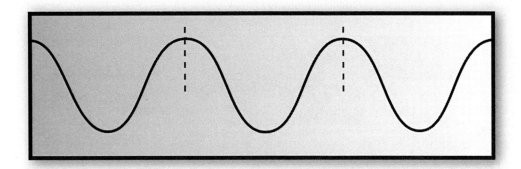

The length of 1 nanometer is 1 billionth of a meter. One thousand nm's equals one micron, which is a millionth of a meter. Thus, a 940 nm laser has a wavelength that is almost one micron. By comparison, the size of this dot (.), used as a period, is about 400 microns or 1/64 inch.

Electromagnetic Spectrum

The diagram on the next page shows the range of emissions called the electromagnetic spectrum. Note that the more damaging emissions, such as x-rays and ultraviolet light, are the shorter wavelengths. The extreme power of these short wavelengths can break the bonds of atoms and produce ions, and for that reason these shorter wavelengths are sometimes called ionizing radiation. Typically, at the other end of the spectrum, radiation in the infrared or visible red spectrum does not cause ionization, but it does generate heat when absorbed in tissue.

Water has very high absorption for light in wavelengths longer than 1500 nm and since water is the major constituent of muscle tissue, this radiation does not penetrate significantly below the skin. We thus are left with an optimum treatment window which is the optical window, between approximately 600 nm to 900 nm where the radiation does not cause ionization and can penetrate beneath the skin to affect the underlying tissue. This is well visualized in the chart below. In the field of low level laser therapy, we use the term optical window to describe the range of 600–900 nm, because lasers that have a wavelength greater than 900 nm produce a lot of heat and are more uncomfortable than the lasers of shorter wavelengths with the same output power.

Note in the diagram below that light in the 600-900 nm wavelength is in the "optical window." This range of wavelengths is most likely to penetrate deeply into the tissues because the photons are not strongly absorbed by hemoglobin or water. When light is absorbed by hemoglobin and water it will be absorbed in the circulatory system and prevented from deeper penetration.

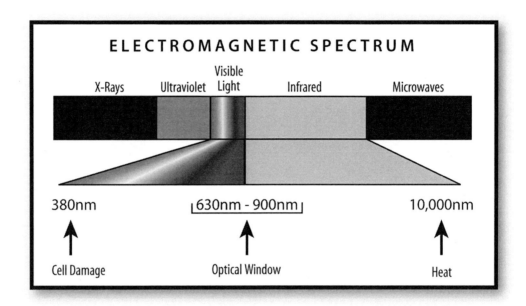

Depth of Laser Penetration

The accepted depth of penetration of a laser depends on its wavelength, but, on average, penetrates about 5–7 cm (2–3+ in.). The majority of photons are absorbed in the first few millimeters. As the laser beam passes into the body, more superficial tissues absorb most of the photons, thus reducing the number of photons that reach deeper layers. However, as these photons enter the body, they create a powerful physiological effect by inducing local metabolic changes and the creation of second messengers. Second messengers are molecules that relay signals received at receptors on the cell surface that target molecules in the nucleus of the cell to modify physiological and genetic information.

Second messengers also serve to greatly amplify the strength of the signal, causing massive changes in the biochemical activities within the cell. Thus, as the effect of the photons diminishes with increasing depth, the physiological effects rapidly multiply, creating a profound and systemic effect. This is how photons quickly create systemic effects.

It was Mester's experiments in 1966–67 that first documented the widespread, systemic effect of laser therapy.

In general, it is well accepted that longer wavelengths, such as 800–900 nm, penetrate slightly deeper than shorter wavelengths, such as 600–700 nm. However, these differences are small and can be overcome by power. For example, a 1,000 mW, 700 nm laser will provide faster, deeper treatment than a 100 mW, 900 nm laser. Thus, it is most important, when choosing a laser or LED device, to balance wavelength and power.

Lasers are more deeply penetrating, but LEDs are less expensive, slightly more superficial, and are very effective when used in unattended LED pads or large laser clusters.

Common Types of Laser Diodes

The wavelength of laser emission is based on the type of diode used in each laser. A diode is created by using a crystal which can be made of various chemicals that cause light to be emitted at a specific wavelength. Gallium-Aluminum-Arsenide (GaAlAs) lasers are the most popular diodes used by laser manufacturers because of their wide range of therapeutic applications and competitive price. Based on the exact structure and composition of the laser, visible red diodes in the 630 to 670 nanometer range and infrared diodes in the 700 to 1000 nm can be made. The shorter wavelength, red diodes are generally much lower power than the longer wavelength, infrared diodes. There are other powerful lasers such as Argon, NdYAG, CO_2, and others that are excellent for surgical and cosmetic use.

Important Terms and Parameters

1. Treatment time is expressed in seconds (sec). This is the most important parameter because it determines total dose.

2. Power is expressed in milliwatts (mW) or Watts (W). 1,000 mW is one Watt. The terms 1,000 milliwatts and 1 Watt are interchangeable.

3. Total dose or energy is expressed in joules (J). This is the power multiplied by the time, Watts x seconds.

4. Wavelength is expressed in nanometers (nm).

5. Frequency is expressed in Hertz (Hz) or cycles per second.

6. Spot size or area is expressed in cm^2.

7. Duty cycle is the percentage of time the light source is ON during one cycle.

8. Power Density or Intensity is expressed in W/cm^2. This is the power divided by the probe size.

9. Energy Density or Fluence is expressed in J/cm^2. This is the total energy delivered divided by the probe size.

Classification of Laser Diodes by Power

Class 4 - More than 500 mW with a collimated beam

These lasers have the potential to cause burns and injuries to the eyes or skin when excessive dose is used. Protective eyewear and strict safety precautions are necessary with Class 4 lasers.

Class 3B – From 5 mW to 500 mW

These lasers can produce eye injuries if looked at directly, but diffuse radiation is considered safe. Protective goggles or glasses are recommended. A collimating lens will increase risk.

Class 3R - Up to 5 mW

Not hazardous if viewed momentarily without protective goggles, especially when the emission has a divergent beam. 3R is limited to 5 mW.

Class 2 or 2M - Up to 1 mW

All Class 2 lasers are considered safe for momentary viewing.

Class 1 or 1M - Less than 1 mW

These lasers present no danger to eye or skin. They are used in many home appliances such as laser printers and other machines where the laser is often not visible and presents no risk of any kind. The beam generally is not collimated.

Light Energy Expressed in Joules

Light energy is expressed in joules (J). This energy is the result of multiplying the number of watts by the treatment time expressed in seconds.

Energy (joules) = Power (Watts) x Time (Seconds)

Some scientists describe a joule as a "Watt-Second," signifying that the number of watts multiplied by the number of seconds is the output in joules. Therefore:

1. A 2,000 mW Laser (2 Watt) applied for 60 seconds, delivers 120 joules of energy.
    a. 2 W x 60 secs = 120 joules

2. A 1,000 mW Laser (1 Watt) applied for 60 seconds, delivers 60 joules of energy.
    a. 1 W x 60 secs = 60 joules

3. A 500 mW (.5W) laser would deliver 30 joules of energy in 60 seconds.
    a. 0.5W x 60 secs = 30 joules

4. A 250 mW (.25W) laser would produce 15 joules of energy in 60 seconds.
    a. 0.25W x 60 secs = 15 joules

Pulsing or Frequency

With the typical low power laser, the frequency is simply the result of turning the beam of light on and off quickly so it flashes or pulses like a strobe light. The typical laser treatment device has a 90% duty cycle meaning that it is ON 90% of the time and OFF 10% of the time. When laser manufacturers state that a laser has a frequency of 1,000 Hertz (Hz), that means that the energy cycles on and off 1,000 times per second and typically has a 90% duty cycle. In the example below, we can see that there is 1 pulse per second or a 1 Hz frequency.

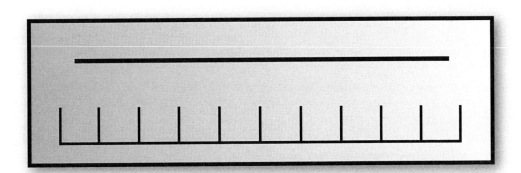

In the above diagram each section is 1/10 of a second and the whole cycle is 1 sec.

In the diagram below, the light is modulated or pulsed at 10 cycles per second or 10 Hz.

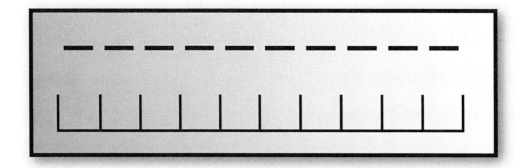

The light in laser treatments does not have to be pulsed. When not pulsed the frequency is called continuous or, cw, for continuous wave. Note that in the example below, the wave is continuous and not pulsed.

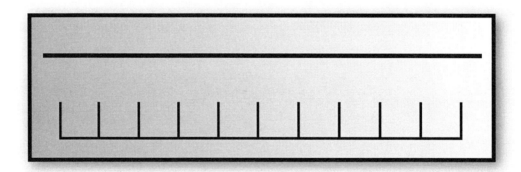

Pulsation is a Natural Part of Life

The earth's surface and the ionosphere produce electromagnetic pulsations of 0.1–25 Hz, with most of the energy being at approximately 10 Hz. We also know that organisms respond to these pulsations with metabolic changes.

We know that pulsing energy can have a physiological effect. However, the exact type of effect that this will produce is presently inconclusive. The simple conclusion is that we do not know whether any treatment frequency is superior to continuous photon emission. Nonetheless, we will list some commonly accepted treatment frequencies, as they are part of many popular protocols.

Treatment Parameters

The following pulse rates are commonly recommended frequencies for various syndromes by a wide variety of authors and manufacturers. It's evidenced by this simple chart that there does not seem to be much agreement about the ideal frequency for any specific condition. Except for Nerve Regeneration and Ligament Repair, the variation is quite wide. This chart helps clarify the poorly understood role played by pulsed operation.

Acute Musculoskeletal	2.5 Hz - 20 Hz
Chronic Musculoskeletal	5 Hz - 150 Hz
Body and Earth Pulsation	1 Hz - 25 Hz
Chronic Pain	2.5 Hz - 150 Hz
Wounds	20 Hz - 5 kHz
Nerve Regeneration	2 Hz
Bone Growth	5 Hz - 10 Hz
Ligament Repair	10 Hz
Granulation Tissue Growth	15, 20, 72 Hz

How Much Light is Absorbed?

It is important that light be applied to clean skin, free from extra oils or creams. Oil will reduce the penetration of the photons by reflecting them off of the skin surface. We have an acronym for how the penetration of photons can occur: "R.A.T.S.," which stands for Reflection, Absorption, Transmission, and Scattering.

As you can see in the diagram below, light will react in varied ways with different types of surfaces and materials. For example, light will reflect off of any oily surface, will be absorbed and transmitted through many cells and will scatter off of metal and plastic implants.

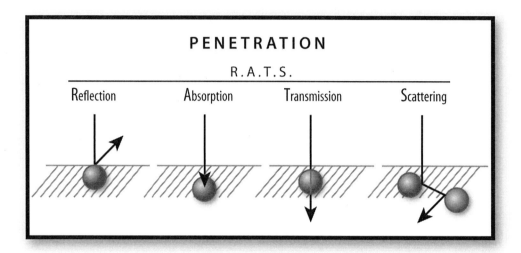

Inverse Square Law

When, during a treatment, the laser or LED is moved away from the skin of the person being treated, the power or dose of the beam will remain constant; however, the intensity or fluence will decrease according to the inverse square law. Assuming that the laser beam is not collimated, the intensity or fluence will decrease proportionally to the increasing area of the beam. If you double the beam diameter by pulling the laser device away from the skin, you reduce the total dose by approximately 1/4.

Ideally, the laser or LED should be applied directly on the skin. If the structure you are treating is buried deep beneath adipose tissue, pressure should be applied to the probe to increase the depth of contact and move the beam closer to the area being treated. This also displaces fluids, such as blood, preventing too many of the photons from being absorbed on their way to the desired tissue. However, when treating wounds to prevent contamination, keep the probe about 1/4 to 1/2 inch above the skin.

SOAP Notes

Good note taking is important in any medical treatment. Always note the Subjective, Objective, Assessment, and Planning information in your daily notes.

Subjective stands for the patient's symptoms, Objective describes any objective observations and/or orthopedic testing, Assessment is the patient's diagnosis or response to treatment, and Plan refers to your treatment plan or what therapy was provided. In the treatment Plan you can note the following factors:

1. NECESSARY: Treatment time in seconds. This is the most important parameter to note as it determines the total dose, since typically the probe power is fixed.

2. NECESSARY: The anatomical location treated.

3. NECESSARY: Total output power of your probe in mW or W. If you only use one probe, this would be optional since you only have one laser instrument.

4. NECESSARY: Wavelength of your probe. If you only use one probe, this would again be optional.

5. OPTIONAL: The total dose or energy in joules. This can be calculated based on treatment time.

6. OPTIONAL: The frequency noted as a pulsed or continuous setting. This can be noted if you use a pulsed treatment modality.

7. OPTIONAL: Power density of your probe. This is used in research studies or if different probe apertures are used. This is not commonly needed in a clinical setting.

Arndt-Schultz Law

The Arndt-Schultz Law describes the relationship between a stimulus or dose and the physiological reaction of the patient. It states the following parameters:

1. A weak stimulus will often elicit a strong reaction.

2. A medium stimulus can cause a moderate reaction.

3. A moderately strong stimulus usually slightly inhibits the system.

4. A very strong stimulus can strongly inhibit the system.

In medicine, when using drug therapy, it is vital to use the ideal dose to achieve a specified effect. A dose above an ideal threshold is called an overdose, will not produce the desired effect and can be toxic. A dose that is too low will not have sufficient power to cause the desired therapeutic effect. In laser and light therapy, the same principles apply. For the most effective laser therapy treatments, one should always use a lower dosage to begin treatment and then titrate up in dose by slightly increasing it on each treatment until the desired effect occurs.

Titration is important because, based on the above principles, providing too much light will inhibit the potential healing effects of laser therapy. This is exemplified by how laser is used in laser surgery where high doses are used to destroy, rather than stimulate tissue.

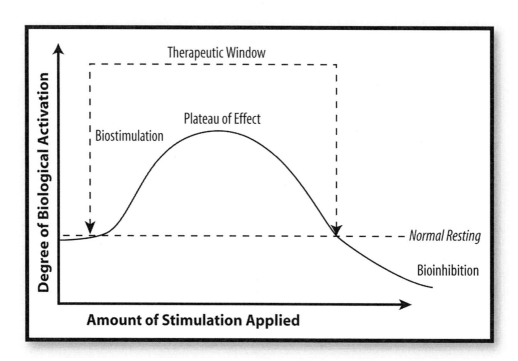

Laser Safety

When one thinks about a laser, one imagines a powerful and narrow "Star Wars" type of beam. Most low level lasers are in the infrared wavelength, so their beam tends to be invisible, increasing the risk of eye injury in the more powerful or highly collimated surgical lasers. However, in the case of Low Level Lasers, the more powerful ones have a divergent beam and a visible red warning light to limit the risk of eye damage.

There are still a number of safety precautions to consider with a laser:

1. Check national, state, and local laws before using your laser or LED.

2. Never look directly into the beam.

3. Make direct contact with the skin at all times or be as close as possible.

4. Have a special treatment room if you are using a hot, Class 4 collimated laser.

5. Turn the laser off before removing it from the skin when you finish a treatment.

6. Practitioner and patient should wear protective goggles during all treatments if you use a hot, collimated, Class 4 laser. However, most practitioners who use a Low Level Laser that is not collimated, with a divergent low power beam, are not required to wear goggles as they do not look directly into the beam during treatment.

Contraindications of Light Therapy

Outside of the precautions regarding eye safety, there are a number of other precautions or contraindications. In spite of the fact that we have no documented evidence that the following problems will occur, it is better to be safe than sorry.

1. Do not treat over a known or suspected tumor or skin cancer. Although there has been no proof that this is dangerous, we do know that laser therapy can stimulate the growth of many types of cells. However, in the field of oncology, laser therapy is being used with many types of cancer patients to help manage pain and oral mucositis. If you are not sure if laser is appropriate, ask the patient's oncologist or physician.

2. Be cautious or avoid treatment during pregnancy. There has been no proof that laser poses danger to pregnancy or pregnant women. Yet, due to the delicate nature of pregnancy and the natural possibilities for spontaneous abortion, a practitioner would be wise to avoid the use of laser during pregnancy.

3. Photosensitivity reactions can occur because of many drugs, including antibiotics such as tetracycline, Retin-A, St. John's Wort, some thyroid medications, and possibly any medication with a warning to avoid bright sunlight. The Skin Patch Test described later in this chapter can be used when a patient is taking any of these medications.

4. Some practitioners believe that laser should not be applied over the thyroid gland because iodine in the thyroid is a strong photo-absorber and could be stimulated by the laser. However, research indicates that low doses are quite safe.

5. Be cautious when treating over tattoos because dark-colored tattoos will absorb light and could become hot and painful.

6. Never treat directly over a bacterial infection. If you are treating an infected wound make sure the patient is on antibiotics and being monitored by a physician.

7. Do not treat patients on immune suppressant drugs since light therapy can stimulate the immune system and possibly interfere with the medical treatment.

9. Be careful treating children or sensitive adults. Always start with a very small total dose such as 25–50 joules for the first treatment.

10. Suspend therapy if the patient feels pain, weakness, or presents any other unusual reaction.

Thermal Damage and Skin Patch Test

It is rare to ever see skin injury after light therapy, but a mild erythematic or a vesicular eruption can occur in photosensitive patients. If in doubt, a small patch test can be carried out prior to full treatment.

Skin Patch Test

1. To perform the Skin Patch Test, apply 10–25 joules of emission to a spot on the arms or legs.

2. If, after waiting approximately five minutes, the patient shows no sign of a negative reaction, then it is often safe to continue with therapy.

3. In cases when extreme caution seems appropriate, such as with chronic pain, highly photosensitive patients, or any unusual medical syndrome, wait 24 hours after a patch test before assessing whether or not the patient is appropriate for therapy.

General Treatment Parameters

The treatment frequency or dose of treatment for Neuromusculoskeletal (NMS) syndromes and wounds depends on the severity of the syndrome. More acute problems require more frequent treatments. With chronic problems, the initial treatment needs a slightly lower dose than for acute injuries, and then also requires less frequent therapy:

Acute Syndromes: Treat 2 to 3 times per week until symptoms subside.

Subacute or Chronic Syndromes: Start with 2 times per week, followed by 1 to 2 times per week until symptoms have resolved.

Minimizing Adverse Side Effects:
The 100 Joule Rule

Excessive laser dosage can cause an adverse response.

1. If you are treating a very healthy, adult patient, the total treatment dose for the first session should not exceed 100 joules. With a high powered, hot laser, this may increase to 200 joules.

2. If the patient is suffering from any type of serious disorder, such as a non-healing wound or chronic pain, it is recommended that the first session utilize no more than 25 joules.

Treating Children: 50 Joule Rule

Use lower power and smaller doses when treating children. It is recommended that when treating children below the age of 12 years, to use an output of 50 joules or less during the first treatment, with a maximum of 50–200 joules or one-third to one-half the adult dosage, based on body weight.

Maximum Dose Depends on Power

1. Lower power lasers (5 to 50 mW) require less total joules per treatment because they are more efficient and a higher percentage of the photons are absorbed by the tissues.

2. Higher power lasers (1,000–20,000 mW) require more total joules because the large number of photons can produce heat and many of the photons are not utilized therapeutically.

3. LEDs require a higher dose because they are not as bright as lasers.

4. Chart A on the following page displays the approximate amount of time necessary to deliver a specific number of joules, based upon the output power 2000 mW. Notice that it takes much longer to achieve a dose between approximately 150–240 joules, a typical full body dose, as the probe output power goes from 1600 mW to 1,000 mW and lower.

Chart A. Time to Deliver Approximately 200 Joules, Based on Probe Output

10,000mW	5000mW	2000mW	1000mW	500mW	100mW	10mW	time (min)
600 J	300 J	120 J	60 J	30 J	6.0 J	0.6 J	1
1200 J	600 J	240 J	120 J	60 J	12 J	1.2 J	2
1800 J	900 J	360 J	180 J	90 J	18 J	1.8 J	3
2400 J	1200 J	480 J	240 J	120 J	24 J	2.4 J	4
3000 J	1500 J	600 J	300 J	150 J	30 J	3.0 J	5
6000 J	3000 J	1800 J	600 J	300 J	60 J	6.0 J	10
9000 J	4500 J	900 J	900 J	450 J	90 J	9.0 J	15
12000 J	6000 J	2400 J	1200 J	600 J	120 J	12 J	20

5.   Chart B below demonstrates how lower power lasers can require less total joules for relief but require more total treatment time. It should be obvious that even achieving an adequate analgesic dose requires a significantly longer time with a low power laser. That is why most practitioners are moving toward more powerful lasers between 500 to 10,000 mW for pain relief.

Chart B. Probe Power and Time to Achieve Pain Relief

Probe Output (mW)	Joules	Minutes
10	9 - 18	15 - 30
100	48 - 90	8 - 12
500	75 - 150	2.5 - 5
1000	120-240	2 - 4
2000	180-360	1.5 - 3
3000	180 - 450	1 - 2
4000	240 - 480	1 - 2
6000	270 - 540	.75 - 1.5
10,000	300 - 600	.5 - 1

Note: This is based solely upon discussions with clinicians who utilize a wide variety of probes and from discussions with manufacturers. The dose noted is based on one or all of the following factors:

1.   The treatment time necessary to consistently create noticeable localized pain relief;

2.   A significant improvement in symptoms such as spasm or loss of range of motion;

3. The maximum treatment dose to achieve a positive effect without creating a flare-up of symptoms.

If you feel that these numbers do not reflect your experience please contact the author through email with your suggested dosage modification. In future editions of this book, these numbers will change based on feedback from clinicians.

Chart C. WALT Recommended Anti-Inflammatory Dosage for Low Level Laser Therapy

Laser Classes 3 or 3 B, 780 - 860nm GaAlAs Lasers. Continuous or Pulse Output less than 0.5 Watt

TENDINOPATHIES	Points or cm²	Joules 780 - 820nm	Notes
Carpal-Tunnel	2 - 3	12	Minimum 6 joules/point
Lateral Epicondylitis	1 - 2	4	Maximum 100mW/cm²
Biceps Humeri c.l.	1 - 2	8	
Supraspinatus	2 - 3	10	Minimum 5 joules/point
Infraspinatus	2 - 3	10	Minimum 5 joules/point
Trochanter Major	2 - 4	10	
Patellartendon	2 - 3	6	
Tract. Iliotibialis	2 - 3	3	Maximum 100mW/cm²
Achilles Tendon	2 - 3	8	Maximum 100mW/cm²
Plantar Fasciitis	2 - 3	12	Minimum 6 joules/point
ARTHRITIS	Points or cm²	Joules 780 - 820nm	Notes
Finger PIP or MCP	1 - 2	6	
Wrist	2 - 4	10	
Humeroradial Joint	1 - 2	4	
Elbow	2 - 4	10	
Glenohumeral Joint	2 - 4	15	Minimum 6 joules/point
Acromioclavicular	1 - 2	4	
Temporomandibular	1 - 2	6	
Cervical Spine	2 - 4	15	Minimum 6 joules/point
Lumbar Spine	2 - 4	40	Minimum 8 joules/point
Hip	2 - 4	40	Minimum 8 joules/point
Knee Medial	3 - 6	20	Minimum 5 joules/point
Ankle	2 - 4	15	

Note: If one compares Chart B and the WALT Chart C, you can observe that when using lower power lasers, in the range of 10–250 mW, the doses in the charts are similar. Note that the WALT Chart C is for treating one area and Chart B is for treating one or more areas, which is not uncommon with a typical patient. Thus, if you treat two or more areas on each patient, the doses are similar.

Symptoms of Excessive Treatment

If the dose is too high, the patient may exhibit any of the following symptoms:

1. Muscular tightness

2. Mild fatigue or nausea

3. Pain at the treatment site

4. Headache

5. An increase in symptom severity

These symptoms can occur during or after treatment and typically last from 1 to 48 hours.

Initial Treatment: 50% Rule

Assuming you are using a 1,000 mW probe, it is safest to start an adult with no more than 100 joules on the first session and for a child, 50 joules. This dose can be increased as long as each successive dose is increased by no more than 50% each treatment. Thus, for adults, the first session would be 100 joules, the next session 150, etc. Obviously, this can be modified depending on the type of patient and/or condition.

See the section on page 32, Dark and Light Skin, for more information on how different variables can affect the first and subsequent doses. It is best to warn the patient of the possibility of some increase in discomfort, even though that is rare.

Optimal Dose for Each Patient

The optimal dose for each patient can vary. This can be judged in the following way:

1. Ask the patient to report any sensation during treatment.

2. A warming or tingling sensation or a lessening of the symptoms can be good signs.

3. An immediate increase in pain is a bad sign. Stop treatment immediately.

4.   Look for an observable reduction in any swelling or inflammation.

5.   Test the patient for improvement in functional capacity.

6.   Palpate the treated area for reduced tenderness and increased tone.

Ask the patient to note and report back any negative reactions or improvements in the 24-hour period following treatment.

Where to Start

Treat from proximal to distal, from the center of the body toward the periphery.

Stimulating the body's central processes will aid treatments to peripheral areas. For example, with lymphedema, stimulating the proximal regions of the leg will increase its physiological activity and prepare it for the increased fluids which will flow up the leg from peripheral treatments to the foot or foreleg. The same is true with manual lymph drainage, it is important to stimulate the proximal leg veins before sending more lymph into them from the foot and ankle.

How Much Time to Spend on Each Region

You will need to decide on your strategy prior to starting laser therapy. In general, it is easy to think about dividing up a treatment session into quarters or thirds.

•   If you have a 2000 mW laser (producing 120 joules per minute) and your treatment times are 2–4 minutes, you might divide the time into thirds. Thus, each treatment portion would be 30–60 seconds for that particular anatomical region.

Treatment By Thirds and Fourths

For example, if someone has a herniated lumbar disc with radiating pain into the foot, you could divide the treatment into fourths:

> One fourth of the time: Treat the disc and nerve roots
> One fourth of the time: Trace the sciatic nerve into the buttocks
> One fourth of the time: Trace the sciatic nerve into the ankle
> One fourth of the time: Treat the ankle and foot

Or, if someone has a herniated lumbar disc with radiating pain into the foot, you could divide the treatment into thirds:

> One third of the time: Treat the disc and nerve roots
> One third of the time: Trace the sciatic nerve into the knee
> One third of the time: Trace the sciatic nerve into the ankle and foot

With carpal tunnel syndrome, you could divide the treatment into fourths:

> One fourth of the time: Treat the trigger points from the elbow toward the wrist
> One fourth of the time: Treat directly over the carpal tunnel
> One fourth of the time: Trace the median nerve from the wrist to the palm
> One fourth of the time: Treat the fingers and fingernails

Or, with carpal tunnel syndrome, you could divide the treatment into thirds:

> One third of the time: Treat the trigger points from the elbow toward the wrist
> One third of the time: Treat directly over the carpal tunnel
> One third of the time: Trace the median nerve from the wrist to the palm

Whether you divide your treatments into thirds or quarters depends on the nature of the patient's syndrome. If the syndrome is simple, such as a bruised quadriceps, you might choose to only divide the treatment time into halves. One half of the time is spent directly over the bruise and one half is spent painting over a larger surrounding area to stimulate adjacent vascular and tissue structures. However, even with a sprained finger, you could divide it up into fourths if you decide to treat all four sides of the joint.

Calculating the Output of Your Probe in Joules

The following is the approximate delivered dose in joules per minute, based on the output power of the probe.

10,000 mW	=	600 joules / minute
5000 mW	=	300 joules / minute
3000 mW	=	180 joules / minute
2000 mW	=	120 joules / minute
1000 mW	=	60 joules / minute
500 mW	=	30 joules / minute
100 mW	=	6 joules / minute
10 mW	=	.6 joules / minute

Maximum Treatment Time

Your total treatment time will be dependent on the strength of your laser because treatment time is inversely proportional to the laser's total output power. The maximum recommended dose for the average patient is 100 to 600 joules, with a probe that is 1,000 to 10,000 mW. Although there are exceptions, mentioned in the clinical part of this manual, we will use that maximum dose for the calculations below:

A 10,000 mW laser will produce 600 joules per minute.

10 watts × 60 seconds = 600 joules per minute

Maximum treatment time: .5–2 minutes depending on the condition

A 5000 mW laser would produce 300 joules per minute.

5 watts × 60 seconds = 300 joules per minute

Maximum treatment time: 1–3 minutes depending on the condition

A 1000 mW laser would produce approximately 60 joules per minute.

1 × 60 seconds = 60 joules per minute

Maximum treatment time: 2–10 minutes depending on the condition

Light Before Heat and After Ice

Because photons are absorbed by blood and water, diminishing their depth of penetration, it is recommended that you use laser and light therapy before any heat and after ice. Because diathermy, ultrasound, and hot packs increase local blood flow, they would also increase local hemoglobin concentration, thus robbing the deeper structures of some photons.

Dark and Light Skin: The 25% Rule

Dark-skinned individuals have more melanin, the brown pigment that blocks out the sun. People from areas farther from the equator have lighter skin and those from the tropics have darker skin. It has been hypothesized that people who live in dark climates might have developed lighter-colored, more translucent skin, in order to help them absorb more of the sun's rays and therefore produce adequate amounts of vitamin D. It has been established that darker-skinned people are blessed with greater natural protection from the harmful sun rays and have a lower risk of skin cancer.

If you are striving for deep laser penetration, it is important to increase the laser dose for a dark-skinned individual and decrease the dose by the same amount when treating a light-skinned individual. The more extreme the skin color, the more you will need to modify your dose.

However, if you are treating superficial tissues, such as the skin itself or acupoints, which lie in the more superficial parts of the ear, then a darker-skinned individual would actually absorb more photons and the dose could be reduced by 25 to 50%.

Thick and Thin Skin

Thick skin is present on the soles of the feet and the palms of the hands. The thicker the skin, the more photons will be required to penetrate the tissue. Thicker skin has a larger stratum corneum with higher keratin content. Thicker skin is observed in scleroderma, progressive systemic sclerosis, and in some patients with insulin-dependent diabetes mellitus. By contrast, aging and some diseases will cause thinning of the skin. Ehlers-Danlos is a syndrome characterized by joint hypermobility and thin, velvety skin. The thinner and whiter the skin, the more the patient will absorb photons and the lower the initial dose will have to be.

A muscular African football player, whose skin feels thick, rough, and calloused, would require a higher dosage. Or, you might find yourself treating a thin, sensitive northern European woman, with Ehlers-Danlos syndrome, who describes herself as being a "sensitive" individual. In both cases, you will need to radically alter your treatment protocols by increasing or decreasing the total dose of therapy accordingly.

Painting and Grid Techniques

Painting:

This technique involves moving a cluster probe with a diameter of 2–5 cm (1–2 inches) over the selected area of treatment about half the speed of ultrasound, or about one inch (2.5 centimeters) every 2 seconds. The movement should be steady, to allow for well-distributed photoabsorption.

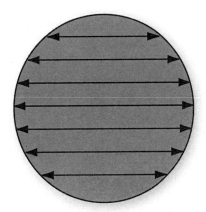

Grid Treatment:

This technique is used when the practitioner uses a point probe that is approximately 1–2 mm in diameter. It is more accurate than scanning and is often used during research or for treating trigger or acupoints. Visualize an imaginary grid of 1 cm (1/2 inch) of intersecting lines over the selected treatment area. The laser tip is applied to each intersecting point of the grid. Although this is an excellent and accurate technique for research, it can be time consuming in daily practice. That is why more practitioners are choosing powerful cluster probes that permit the use of the painting techniques.

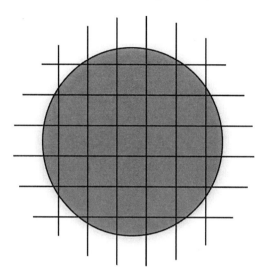

Quick Scan: Easy Treatment for Chronic Pain

One of the simplest techniques for chronic pain is called the Quick Scan. It is based on the premise that photons should be delivered primarily to the site of injury. It also assumes that stimulating along the transverse processes of the spine, above the sympathetic chain, can create a feeling of relaxation and help reduce global pain perception. If there is any pain that radiates down the arm or leg, treatment of the ipsilateral finger or toe nails, because they are translucent, may help stimulate the involved peripheral nerves. Thus, the protocol would be divided into thirds:

1. Treat the site of pain for one-third of the total treatment time.

2. Treat along the transverse processes of the spine from C7 to L2, to stimulate the sympathetic chain ganglia, for one-third of the time.

3. Treat the finger or toe nails of the ipsilateral side of injury for the remainder of the allotted treatment time.

Nerve Tracing

Nerve tracing is used in cases with neuritis, sciatica, and radiculopathy. It involves palpation along the skin overlaying the tract of a peripheral nerve, looking for sore, tender points. Often the tender point is slightly raised, possibly indicating increased muscle tonus. The protocol would be:

1. Trace the nerve from proximal to distal.

2. Palpate the skin over a nerve looking for tender or swollen points.

3. Treat the most important tender points.

Hot and Cold Imbalance

1. Stimulation of a cooler region with light can create increased warmth; stimulating a warmer region can create increased coolness.

2. This occurs because light has the ability to both stimulate and alter the autonomic nervous system, therefore stimulating natural homeostasis.

Relaxation Technique

1. When the probe is placed against the skin you will feel a certain amount of tissue resistance.

2. As you provide light or laser stimulation you will, at some point, feel the probe gently sink into the tissue.

3. This may reflect a relaxation response by the connective tissue.

4. This often means that the patient has received sufficient stimulation to relax tissues and is a sign to stop treatment on that particular point or region.

How to Choose the Right Device for Your Practice

Whether you choose a laser or an LED device, it is important to remember that the treatment time is inversely proportional to the total power output. Thus, a 1,000 mW laser will require approximately half the treatment time of a 500 mW laser.

In general, LEDs require longer treatment times than a laser because they are not as bright and have lower intensity. If you want the power of a 1,000 mW laser on an LED device, it would be wise to purchase a 2,000 mW LED to achieve similar effects. The following are general guidelines when choosing a laser or light therapy device.

1. If you primarily treat musculoskeletal conditions, large animals, and only occasionally treat wounds, it might make sense to purchase an infrared laser probe of 500 mW or higher.

2. If you want short treatment times of 1–2 minutes and want to easily treat the entire body, including odd-shaped surfaces such as the knee and ankle, choose a laser between 1,000–10,000 mW.

3. If you do not want to spend a lot of time treating patients but want a low cost device, consider purchasing a powerful LED. They are excellent when unattended therapy is required and they are now being made in a wide variety of sizes and shapes, for different body parts.

4. If the focus of your practice is treating wounds and skin conditions, consider a mixed visible red and infrared LED probe, since deep penetration will not be needed and red lasers are very costly. However, an infrared laser also works very well for wounds and superficial conditions.

5. If you treat acupuncture points or practice auriculotherapy, consider purchasing a small infrared or red laser point probe with 50 to 500 mW.

6. If you are primarily concerned about creating analgesia, you can use a high power laser with 5,000–10,000 mW or use a 1,000–5,000 mW LED.

Power Density or Intensity

We know that a 1,000 mW laser produces 60 joules for every minute of treatment. However, the density of the power output will vary depending on the size of the head of the probe. For example, a 1,000 mW laser that is 1 inch (2.5 cm) in diameter will have a lower power density than a 1,000 mW head that is 1/10 of an inch (2.5 mm). This works similarly to the water pressure through a shower or a hose: When you make the stream of water narrower in a shower or garden hose, you are increasing the power density of that stream although you are generally not changing the amount of total water flowing through the system. This understanding of power density is important because it will help you choose the probe needed for a specific type of treatment.

Acupuncture laser probes are often very small and provide more power in a smaller area (since acupuncture points are small). Probes for treating large wounds and broad muscular areas are wider because it is easier to "sweep" or "paint" an area than to move a small point probe over a large number of discrete, tiny points. Thus, a 1,000 mW acupuncture probe and a 1,000 mW laser or LED cluster would provide the exactly same amount of joules per minute, but the density of the stream would be much more intense with the smaller-aperture acupuncture (point) probe.

To calculate Power Density or Intensity, you only need to know the total power output of your probe or pad in Watts or Milliwatts and the size of the aperture or treating surface of the probe.

$$\text{Power density} = \frac{\text{Power in Watts or Milliwatts}}{\text{Spot Size or Surface Area in cm}^2}$$

To compute the surface area or spot size of your probe, you can use the equation:

Surface Area of a probe = $\pi \times r^2$ (π is 3.14, r is the radius of the probe in cm)

Surface Area of a pad = length of pad $\times$ width of pad

In either case you would divide the total number of mW or W by the surface area in cm^2.

Calculation of Power Density

Let's compare the power density of a 1,000 mW, 2 inch diameter cluster and a 1/32 inch point probe with the same output, 1,000 mW.

To calculate this, one needs to find out the surface area of the tip of each probe. A probe usually has a beam that is circular, so the equation used to find out the surface area of a circular probe tip is the equation used to find the area of a circle.

The equation used to find the area of a circle or the area of a probe tip is:

$\pi \times r^2$ = area of a circle
3.14 $\times$ radius^2 in cm = area of the probe tip

Large Musculoskeletal Laser with 1,000 mW

If you have a 5 cm diameter (2 inch) laser probe or LED cluster, the probe tip radius would be half of that or 2.5 cm:

$$3.14 \times 2.5 \text{ cm}^2 = 19.6 \text{ cm}^2$$

If this is a 1,000 mW (1 watt) probe, it would produce 1 watt or 1 joule per second. The power density or intensity is then:

$$1 \text{ Watt} / 19.6 \text{ cm}^2 = 0.051 \text{ W/cm}^2$$

Small Acupuncture Laser or LED point probe with 1,000 mW

If you have a 0.1 cm diameter (1/25 inch) laser probe the probe tip radius would be half of that or .05 cm:

$$3.14 \times 0.05 \text{ cm}^2 = 0.0078 \text{ cm}^2$$

If this is a 1,000 mW (1 watt) probe, it would produce 1 watt or 1 joule per second. The power density or intensity is then:

$$1 \text{ Watt} / 0.0078 \text{ cm}^2 = 127 \text{ W/cm}^2$$

Thus the small acupuncture probe is about 2,500 times more intense than the large musculoskeletal probe!

However, both lasers put out the exact same number of joules each second: each puts out 1,000 mW or 1 watt, so they each produce 1 joule each second.

Thus, both produce 60 joules per minute, even with a dramatically different power density. In general, the treatment time would be the same for both probes because both deliver the same total dose.

What is the difference?

1. If you use the small acupuncture probe, with a high power density, you will need to keep the probe moving more quickly from point to point, to spread out the delivery of photons, than with the larger, less dense cluster.

2. Thus:

   The power density determines treatment technique.

   The output power determines the treatment time.

What does this mean in practical terms?

Generally speaking, pads and probes with lower power densities produce less heat and higher power densities produce more intense heat. What this means in your clinic is that if you have a large LED pad with a low power density, you can leave it on the patient for a longer period of time without worrying about skin burning. If you have a high power density probe, you will need to keep the probe moving to make sure that you do not burn the patient's skin.

Surgical lasers often have dramatically higher total power and power densities than low level or cold lasers. That is what makes the therapy laser so much safer than a surgical laser.

Dose versus Density

It is logical to think that a 100 mW laser used for 60 seconds will have the same effect as 1,000 mW for 6 seconds since they both deliver 6 joules of energy. However, skin irritation or burns can occur, when the intensity or density is very high. That is why most high power laser manufacturers recommend that a clinician keep the probe moving at all times or widen the spot size to lower the power density.

For example, what if we want to bake a chicken? How would temperature change your cooking procedures?

Let's say that you plan to bake your chicken for 60 minutes at 300° F. Would it be different to roast it for 30 minutes at 600° F? Yes, it would! When using a very extreme amount of heat, enough to denature the tissue, the rules will change.

How about 1800° F for 10 minutes? I think that you can see that cooking chicken at 1800° F for 10 minutes would likely burn the outside and produce raw chicken on the inside.

So, the Baked Chicken Principle is that as long as you are using a laser with a diffuse beam, and there is very little heat output, you can assume that your total dose in joules is a reasonable and consistent measurement of how much energy or treatment was provided to a patient.

However, very high-powered lasers that produce a lot of heat do not follow the same principles as diffuse lasers because they can produce tissue destruction and denature the cellular structure of the area being treated.

Dose is a Better Guide than Density

It is easier for the practitioner to use the concept of total joules (dose) than joules/cm^2 (density) because the density can be confusing and lead to inaccurate total dosage.

For example, the diagram below represents a laser or LED probe with a power output of 1,000 mW or 1 W. Assuming that the size of the diode is 1 cm^2, the Power Density is 1 joule per cm^2 (remember that 1 Watt per second is one joule). If this probe was placed on a patient's back, the Total Dose after one minute of treatment is 60 joules.

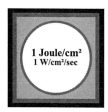

If the practitioner now switches to a much bigger probe head with the same Power Density, but 9 diodes rather than 1 diode, the Power Density is exactly the same, but the dose is 9 times stronger. The 9 diode probe is emitting 9,000 mW and has the exact same Power Density as the probe emitting 1,000 mW!

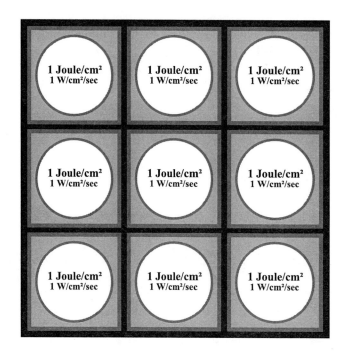

Treatment and Dosage Guidelines

1. For any one anatomical area, the lower dosages are better for stimulating healing and higher dosages will provide more pain relief.

2. The lower end of the range could used be to stimulate healing in one area.

3. For deeper areas, use the longer treatment time in the range but keep the probe moving to avoid overheating and flaring the area.

4. If you want to treat 3 areas, use the lower part of the range, but be careful not to over-treat.

5. With higher power lasers in the range of 5,000–10,000 mW extra caution needs to be exercised when treating multiple areas to avoid flaring up the patient.

You will find these charts at the beginning of each chapter of diagrams on pages 50, 66, 78, 100, and 128.

.

Head & Face
Treatments

Bell's Palsy (diagram page 51, dose page 50)

Subjective: The patient will usually complain of an acute onset of unilateral upper and lower facial paralysis. This may be accompanied by ear pain, decreased hearing, occasionally hyperacusis and taste abnormalities. Onset may be insidious or after infection, trauma, or toxic exposure.

Objective: There is unilateral facial paralysis that corresponds to the course of the seventh cranial (facial) nerve. When the patient is asked to raise the eyebrows or smile, there will be no response on the affected side. In more severe cases, the patient may not be able to close the eye completely on the affected side. Some physicians believe that the cause is inflammation of the facial nerve, a viral infection, or both.

Assessment: The patient will often notice a decrease in discomfort, especially at night, after the first treatment.

Laser Treatment Plan: Treatment can begin two to three times per week as long as symptoms are stable or improving. Begin by painting over the area of palsy as well as the course of the facial nerve with no more than 25 joules. Slowly increase dosage over the course of therapy with a maximum dose of 50 to 600 joules per treatment.

Adjunctive Treatment Plan: The patient should be educated about proper eye care and in facial exercise techniques. Taping the eye shut at night can make sleeping easier and protect the eye from injury.

Migraine Headache (diagrams pages 52–53, dose page 50)

Subjective: Migraine headaches typically start with a prodrome that can be days to minutes prior to the onset of pain. The prodorome will progress to a moderate to severe throbbing sensation, is often unilateral, and is localized to the frontal, temporal and parietal area and can create nausea and vomiting. Over a period of hours, the pain becomes more diffuse and can last from several hours to several days in severe cases. Sensitivity to light and sound is not uncommon.

Objective: History, pain pattern, and response to medication are the most accepted criteria for migraine diagnosis. Imaging studies may be necessary to rule out other causes.

Assessment: A temporary decrease in pain is common with laser therapy. Long lasting cures of migraine with laser therapy have not been documented in research or clinical practice.

Laser Treatment Plan: Begin treating sore acupoints and trigger points with 5 to 25 joules per point, for a maximum of 50–600 joules per session, for 1–2 days to help alleviate symptoms. Laser auriculotherapy may also provide some benefit.

Adjunctive Treatment Plan: Some patients who experience migraines have dietary triggers in chocolate, aged cheese, aged meat, wine, beer and citrus fruits. Other triggers can include heat, stress, and lack of sleep. Meditation, visualization, biofeedback and stress reduction techniques may help patients adapt to the chronic nature of their pain. In moderate to severe cases, medication is usually necessary, although nutritional supplementation and herbal compounds have been shown to be helpful in many cases.

Sinusitis (diagram page 54, dose page 50)

Subjective: Patients usually complain of chronic pain in and around one or more of the four sinuses in the frontal and maxillary bones. There may also be nasal stuffiness, the feeling of facial fullness, dental pain, fever, and ear pain.

Objective: History and physical/manual exam is usually definitive. Occasionally there is a need for x-rays, CT, MRI, or endoscopic culture.

Assessment: There will be a decrease in subjective complaints if inflammation and infection are alleviated.

Laser Treatment Plan: Be certain that there is no infection prior to treating with laser therapy. If there is a significant amount of mucous, ask the patient to consult their doctor or start a saline flush before starting laser therapy. The mucous must be loose and draining before using a laser on the sinuses. Once the sinuses have started to drain, paint over the sinuses, starting with a total of 25–100 joules spread over the problematic sinuses, approximately 2 to 3 times per week. Intraoral irradiation into the maxillary sinus, radiation into the nostrils and treatment between the eyebrows can be of benefit. Only increase the dose if the patient is reporting an improvement in symptoms, and as long as the patient is using a saline wash.

Adjunctive Treatment Plan: Washing the sinuses with saline on a regular basis can be very helpful. Check environmental sensitivities or allergic factors as they may predispose some individuals to this condition. Ask the patient to reduce exposure to dust, molds, cigarette smoke, and irritants. In some cases, adding a mild herbal disinfectant to the saline flush or having a physician prescribe a liquid antibiotic from a compounding pharmacy can produce faster, more effective results.

Temporomandibular Joint (TMJ) Syndrome (diagram page 55, dose page 50)

Subjective: Patients typically complain of pain in and around the TMJ. There is often increased pain with chewing, occasional popping and clicking. Many patients also complain of earache, headache, and limitation of jaw movement.

Objective: Most patients exhibit pain with direct palpation of the TMJ, and may have limitation of jaw opening, and palpable spasm of the masseter and temporalis. Clicking or popping in the TMJ, crepitus, and jaw deviation occur in some cases. If the problem is confined primarily to soft tissue pain, the term TM dysfunction is often used while TMJ syndrome is used when there is objective, visible damage to the joint. Imaging studies are effective in documenting TMJ damage.

Assessment: Improvement is observed as decreased subjective complaints, less muscle spasm, with improving range of jaw motion.

Laser Treatment Plan: Treat the masseter, pterygoids, and temporalis muscles. Rarely does the joint need more than 10 to 100 joules, but the muscles do require a stronger dose. Begin with 25 joules on the first treatment and, with a higher probe, titrate up to a maximum of 600 joules if condition shows improvement with each increase.

Adjunctive Treatment Plan: The use of ice and heat is recommended to control inflammation and pain. Educate the patient about bruxism, tongue and jaw position, and the need to avoid clenching. Stress can play a major role in the disturbance of jaw posture and thus stress reduction strategies and behavior modification can be of benefit. Good posture, soft food and smaller bites can make eating easier. If treatment is ineffective a splint to stabilize the TMJ is another option.

Tension Headache (diagrams pages 52–53, dose page 50)

Subjective: Tension headaches are characterized by a generalized aching that tends to be experienced as a constant pressure in the frontal, temporal, and occipital regions. Many patients state that stress, eyestrain, bad posture, and hunger can aggravate their condition.

Objective: Patients with tension headaches have normal neurologic and orthopedic examination findings. Some patients may have tenderness in the suboccipital and frontal muscles or palpable cervical muscle spasm.

Assessment: Since lab and imaging studies only rule out pathology and are not diagnostic, patient history and pain level are utilized to asses improvement after treatment. Tight muscles in neck and face should decrease.

Laser Treatment Plan: Deliver 25 to 100 joules to the area of discomfort, primarily the suboccipital and upper cervical regions. Follow this with painting of the frontal or temporalis muscles if pain is also present in those regions. Using a point probe to treat acupoints and trigger points may also be of benefit. Apply 5–25 joules per point, and consider 50–600 joules to be an approximate total treatment dose. Focus on the points that exhibit the most discomfort with palpation.

Adjunctive Treatment Plan: The use of ice and heat is recommended to control inflammation and pain. Additional techniques include cervical stretching exercises, massage, ultrasound therapy, and cranial and cervical spine mobilization. Some patients find benefit from meditation, stress management, and biofeedback techniques.

Trigeminal Neuralgia (diagram page 56, dose page 50)

Subjective: Trigeminal neuralgia is characterized by severe bursts of pain in one or more branches of the trigeminal nerve. The bursts are quick, repetitive jabs of pain, irregularly many times a minute. The patient may wince, twitch, or cry out because the pain is excruciating. Trigeminal neuralgia differs from atypical facial pain which is similar but is usually burning, aching, dull, or crushing. Moreover, an atypical facial pain attack usually lasts minutes or hours.

Objective: An MRI scan can be helpful, although most studies will be normal. Referral to a physician is necessary to rule out the possibility of cluster headache, migraine, TMJ pain, atypical facial pain and tumor.

Assessment: Treatment will result in a reduction of pain. Complete pain relief is unlikely if there is direct compression of the trigeminal nerve. Pain due to inflammation of the nerve responds slowly and steadily with increasing treatment.

Laser Treatment Plan: Trace over the symptomatic trigeminal nerve three times per week starting with a total dose of no more than 25 joules and increasing the dosage only if there is no flare-up or some improvement occurs with treatment. Gradually increase the dose and decrease the frequency as symptoms improve. Generally, it is rare that the patient will need more than a total of 50 to 600 joules.

Adjunctive Treatment Plan: Medication, pain management, and surgery can be necessary when pain is intractable. In some cases cranial therapy is very effective.

Wrinkles (dose page 50)

Subjective: Patient presents with a desire for a smoother facial complexion.

Objective: The size and depth of lines can be measured, although typically patients are very aware of their facial contours and can report quite accurately if treatment is making a difference.

Assessment: Patient and therapist can observe a lessened number of the shallower wrinkles.

Laser Treatment Plan: Start treating with 50 to 100 joules the first visit and increase to 200–600 joules if there are no side effects and patient is happy with the results. It could take one to two months of treatment, 2 to 3 times per week, to produce a significant change.

Adjunctive Treatment Plan: Make sure the patient is using a quality moisturizing cream after each treatment. Some therapists report that supplementing the treatment with oral hyaluronic acid and essential fatty acids can increase the speed and quality of improvement.

Head & Face Diagrams

Typical Treatment Time and Joules based on Power of Probe

Probe Output (mW)	Joules	Treatment Time
10	6 - 12	10 - 20 mins
100	36 - 72	6 - 12 mins
500	60 - 180	2 - 6 mins
1,000	90 - 240	1.5 - 4 mins
2,000	120 - 360	1 - 3 mins
3,000	180 - 450	1 - 2.5 mins
4,000	240 - 480	1 - 2 mins
6,000	270 - 540	.75 - 1.5 mins
10,000	300 - 600	.5 - 1 mins

The above chart notes the approximate treatment times based on the power of the probe being used. Since the suggested treatment doses in this book are for LEDs and lasers in the range of 10 to 10,000 mW, full body treatment times will be approximately 1–15 minutes and approximately 100 to 1200 joules. If you are using a lower power laser or LED, you will need to use longer treatment times, and proportionally less joules.

Use this chart as a guide for an approximate treatment time and dosage based on your particular laser or LED and the individual needs of the patient.

Bell's Palsy

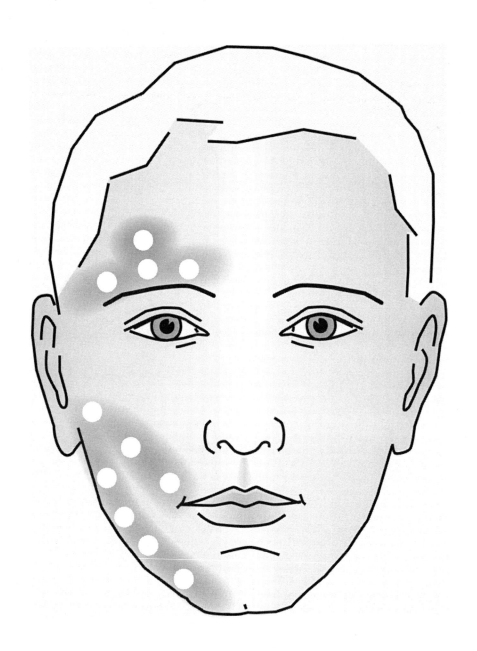

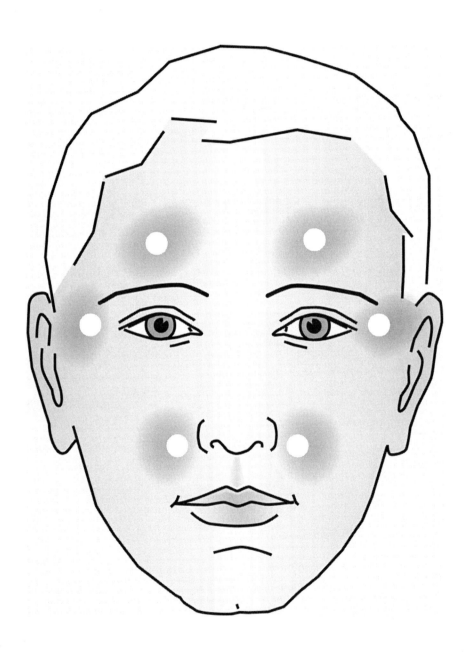

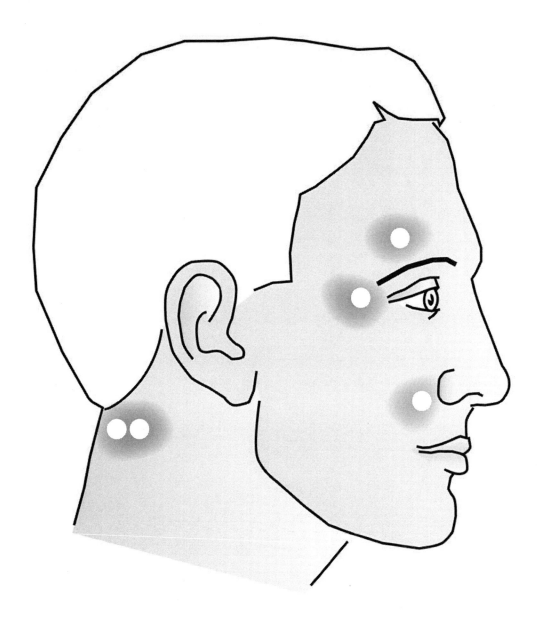

Sinusitis

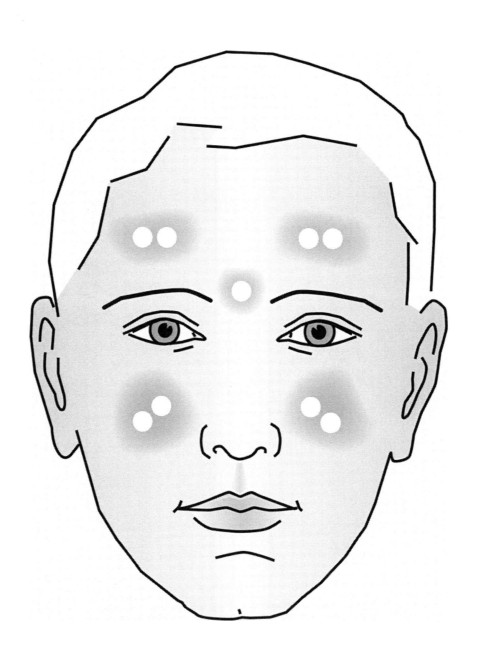

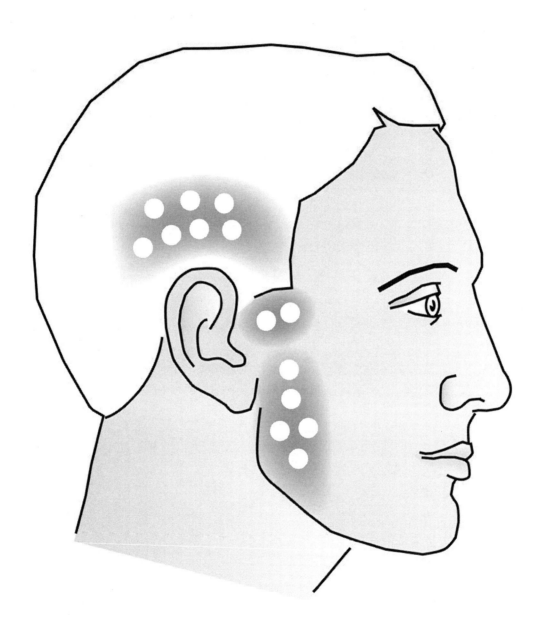

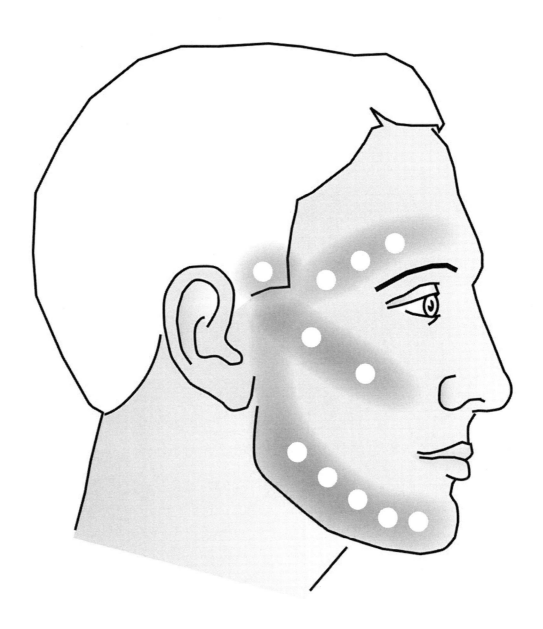

Spine & Pelvis Treatments

Cervical Disc Herniation (diagram page 68, dose page 66)

Subjective: Herniated cervical discs create pain in the lateral neck and shoulder in mild cases. In moderate to serious cases, there can be severe pain that radiates into the ipsilateral middle back, arm and hand. The patient may present a history of trauma, but insidious onset is common.

Objective: These patients often complain of pain with ipsilateral cervical spine side bending that, in more serious cases, radiates into shoulder, middle back, arm and hand. Many patients also increase their pain with cervical extension. In more severe cases, there can be motor weakness and altered reflexes. Often there is some relief when the patient lies supine with the neck in a slightly flexed position and the arm adducted, across the chest or flexed overhead. X-rays are often not useful but can help rule out other causes. MRI and CT scans provide the most information about the severity of the herniation.

Assessment: Improvement will result in centralization of pain followed by decreasing neck pain, increasing range of motion, and, when present, normalizing neurological signs.

Laser Treatment Plan: Treat the site of herniation with 25–600 joules and then slowly paint over the nerve roots in the lateral neck with 10 to 100 joules. Finally, trace a few tender points in the arm with 5 to 25 joules per tender point. Treat two to three times per week for two to six weeks, decreasing frequency as symptoms improve.

Adjunctive Treatment Plan: Most patients find relief from avoiding cervical spine extension and ipsilateral side bending. Many patients report relief from gentle home traction and regular resting in the supine position, to minimize loading of the disc. Prescribe arm and chest stretches to relieve brachial tension, with an emphasis on middle back strengthening as symptoms abate. Initial use of ice and then later use of ice/heat on the cervical spine can be helpful to decrease inflammation and control symptoms. A home program that includes upper extremity stretching can be helpful. If symptoms are not improving after two to three weeks, or if there is increasing pain or motor weakness, consider a referral to an orthopedic specialist.

Cervical Stenosis (diagram page 68, dose page 66)

Subjective: The patient will complain of pain in the lateral neck and shoulder in mild cases. In moderate to severe cases, the pain will radiate into the ipsilateral middle back and arm. The patient will often present with a forward, flexed head position.

Objective: X-rays can be helpful, especially oblique views. MRI and CT scans provide the most information about the severity of the stenosis. There is often increased pain with ipsilateral cervical spine side bending and extension, causing radiating pain into the shoulder, middle back, and/or arm and hand in moderate to severe cases. With more serious cases, there can be motor weakness, decreased range of motion, and altered reflexes.

Assessment: Improvement will result in centralization of pain, followed by decreasing neck symptoms and improved cervical range of motion.

Laser Treatment Plan: Treat the site of stenosis with 25–600 joules and then slowly paint over the nerve roots in the lateral neck with 10 to 100 joules. Finally trace a few tender points in the arm with 5 to 25 joules per tender point. Treat two to three times per week for two to six weeks, decreasing frequency as symptoms improve.

Adjunctive Treatment Plan: Most patients find relief from avoiding cervical spine extension and side bending. Prescribe arm and chest stretches to relieve brachial muscular and nerve tension, with an emphasis on middle back strengthening as symptoms abate. Initial use of ice and then later use of ice/heat on the cervical spine can be helpful to decrease inflammation and control symptoms. A home program that includes application of heat to the arm and upper extremity stretching can be helpful. Some patients find relief from traction, as long it is performed with the neck in a slightly flexed position. If symptoms are not improving after two to three weeks of laser treatment, or if there is increasing pain or motor weakness, consider a referral to an orthopedic/physical medicine specialist or spine surgeon.

Cervical, Thoracic, Lumbar Sprain/Strain and Neuritis (diagram page 67, dose page 66)

Subjective: Sprains and strains typically cause localized back or neck pain. In moderate cases, there will be muscle spasm and even radiating pain into an extremity or around the ribs and into the chest or abdomen, especially with moderate injuries to facets or ribs. The patient may feel relief with flexion or extension.

Objective: There will be pain on palpation with no positive motor or reflex changes. Look for localized stiffness or joint blocking, often accompanied by muscle spasm. Imaging studies are usually negative. In moderate to severe cases, the joint may "click" or "clunk" during activity and you need to examine the patient for joint laxity and hypermobility.

Assessment: With appropriate therapy, the patient will note improved joint play with decreasing spasm and pain within the first few treatments.

Laser Treatment Plan: Treat two to three times the first week, decreasing frequency as symptoms subside. Treat with 10 to 100 joules directly over the problem facet. Treat with 5 to 25 joules per tender point if there is radiating pain down the arm, leg, or along intercostal nerves if there is a radiating neuritis. Maximum initial dose should not exceed 100 to 150 joules, increasing to a maximum of 600 joules per session.

Adjunctive Treatment Plan: In the acute stage, the patient should avoid any position or movement that increases pain. Initially using ice for 2 to 3 days and then ice/heat can assist in symptom control. Mobilization often provides dramatic relief of symptoms. Patient should only perform exercises that provide relief from pain in early stages and progress to gentle stretching and strengthening as symptoms decrease. With rib sprains, no flexion or side-bending stretching should be performed for one to two days after joint mobilization. If one week of treatment has not produced significant improvement, consider referral to an ortho-pedic specialist for more potent anti-inflammatories and an additional diagnostic workup.

Coccydynia (diagram page 68, dose page 66)

Subjective: Patients usually complain of lower coccyx pain that is aggravated by sitting. Although onset can be insidious, the most common cause is direct trauma or repeated strain caused by activities such as cycling or rowing. Childbirth, due to the increased flexibility of the joint and the resulting strain and pressure, can also cause this syndrome. The result is an injury of the sacro-coccygeal junction.

Objective: Physical examination demonstrates that the coccygeal region usually is markedly ten-der to direct palpation. X-rays may reveal a distortion of the normal coccygeal configuration.

Assessment: Improvement will be noted after 1–2 weeks as a decrease in localized, sacrococ-cygeal complaints. If improvement is interrupted by a flare-up, make certain that the patient uses upright and slightly forward leaning posture when sitting.

Laser Treatment Plan: Begin treatment with 25 to 100 joules with half of the treatment painting directly over the sacrococcygeal junction and the other half slowly painting the adjacent areas of the sacrum and gluteal muscles.

Adjunctive Treatment Plan: To reduce direct strain on the coccyx, patients need to be encour-aged to avoid sitting down for long periods of time. Sitting on the edge of the chair, with the weight on the ischial tuberosities, can often reduce pain over time. Some practitioners believe that intra-anal mobilization techniques may be of benefit. Anti-inflammatories, ice, and sitting on a "doughnut" cushion or pillow can help control symptoms. In acute cases a stool softener can reduce discomfort during defecation.

Costochondritis (diagram page 67, dose page 66)

Subjective: This condition often presents with sternal or rib pain localized to the costal cartilage. This syndrome is common after motor vehicle accidents and sports injuries, but can be of insidious onset.

Objective: There is pain on palpation over the sternocostal joints and often the more painful joints protrude slightly anterior. There is often a corresponding dysfunction in the vertebral joints in the middle back.

Assessment: Treatment usually results in rapid resolution of the majority of symptoms.

Laser Treatment Plan: Treat each tender sternocostal joint with 10 to 50 joules and then paint over the wider symptomatic area with 25 to 100 joules. Treatment in the acute stage often requires no more than two to five treatments, each with a maximum of 50 to 600 joules.

Adjunctive Treatment Plan: Ice/heat at home can help reduce inflammation. Stretching should be avoided for one to two days after treatment. Gentle mobilization of the sternocostal and costovertebral joints can help alleviate dysfunction, when present.

Herniated Lumbar Disc or Annular Tear

(diagram page 68, dose page 66)

Subjective: A herniated lumbar disc will create low back and/or leg pain that is increased with at least one or two of the following activities: coughing, sneezing, sitting, long term standing, rolling over in bed, moving from lying or sitting to standing, and repeated bending, twisting, and lifting.

Objective: There will often be decreased lumbar range of motion with lumbar muscle spasm, positive sitting straight leg raise, and a positive Valsalva. With moderate to severe injuries there can be sciatica, numbness, tingling, motor and reflex changes. MRI or CT may demonstrate herniation when the protrusion is significant.

Assessment: Proper therapy usually results in improving range of motion, decreased pain, and less positive orthopedic tests.

Laser Treatment Plan: On the first treatment, start with 25–600 joules depending upon the severity of the injury. Always start with a lower dose and titrate upward slowly. Treat two to three times the first week, decreasing frequency as symptoms improve. Use lower doses if patient has severe pain, to reduce the likelihood of a flare-up. Spend one-third of the treatment time directly over the injured disc, one-third painting the lumbar nerve roots above and across the crest of the ilium, and one-third of the dose treating points in the buttocks and leg. Treatment may be required over the lumbar or leg muscles if there is spasm, including hamstrings, quadratus lumborum, gluteus medius, and tensor fascia lata. .

Adjunctive Treatment Plan: In the acute stage, the patient should decrease sitting, bending, twisting, and lifting. Initially using ice and then ice/heat can assist in symptom control. A back brace often provides an increased sense of stability during the most acute stage.

The patient should only perform exercises that provide relief from pain in early stages and progress to stabilization exercises and leg stretching as symptoms decrease. Later, progression to stabilization and strengthening of core muscles is recommended. Traction can be provided when appropriate, and education about posture and body mechanics is vital. If there is no improvement after one to two weeks or symptoms worsen, a referral to an orthopedic specialist may be indicated for an MRI or other types of intervention. If there is bladder or bowel disruption or a noticeable increase in neurological symptoms, especially motor weakness, refer the patient to a physician immediately.

Lumbar Stenosis (diagram page 68, dose page 66)

Subjective: Lumbar stenosis commonly presents with low back pain that radiates into the hip and lower extremity, aggravated by lumbar spine extension. Often lying prone aggravates the pain, while slumped sitting and pelvic tilt positions can give some relief.

Objective: There is moderate or increased pain with lumbar spine extension and, in moderate to severe stenosis, there can be altered reflexes and motor weakness. The stenosis in the central or lateral canal is usually visible on x-ray, MRI, or CT. This syndrome is more common in older people and rare in patients under 50 years old.

Assessment: If treatment is successful, the patient will experience less radiating pain and improved functional activities.

Laser Treatment Plan: Treat the site of stenosis with 25 to 200 joules and then paint over the nerve roots with 10 to 100 joules above the crest of the ilium. Finally, trace the radiating pain down the sciatic nerve with 5 to 25 joules per tender point with treatment of the foot and toenails in severe cases, for a maximum of 50 to 600 joules per session.

Adjunctive Treatment Plan: Initial use of ice and then later use of ice/heat on the lumbar spine can be helpful to decrease inflammation and control symptoms. A home program that includes application of heat to the leg muscles and lower extremity stretching can also be helpful. Most patients find relief from gentle flexion exercises, leg stretches, with an emphasis on abdominal and core strengthening. If symptoms are not improving after two to three weeks, or if there is increasing pain or motor weakness, consider an immediate referral to an orthopedic specialist.

Pubic Symphysis Sprain (diagram page 68, dose page 66)

Subjective: This syndrome will create pain at the pubic symphysis, aggravated by activity, even walking. In more severe cases, patients can hear a "clicking" emanating from the joint with vigorous physical activity, trauma, pregnancy, or obesity.

Objective: There is pain on palpation directly over the symphysis pubis with a palpable asymmetry in the alignment of the pubic bones. There is often a concomitant dysfunction of the sacroiliac joint.

Assessment: With improvement, there is a rapid decrease in subjective complaints.

Laser Treatment Plan: Place the laser directly over the most painful part of the pubic bones for 10 to 100 joules. Then paint over the area with 25 to 50 joules. Treatment can be provided two to three times per week for one to three weeks, decreasing frequency of treatment as symptoms abate. Because the symphysis is close to the genitals, consider having the patient hold the probe over the pubis.

Adjunctive Treatment Plan: Initial use of ice and then later use of ice/heat can be helpful to decrease inflammation and control symptoms. Patients should avoid any extreme range of motion of the lower extremities. Isometric thigh adduction and abduction can strengthen and stabilize the region once the acute symptoms have been relieved. In some cases, mobilization or stabilization of the sacroiliac joint can help alleviate pubic symptoms.

Sacroiliac Sprain or Strain
(diagram page 67, dose page 66)

Subjective: A sacroiliac sprain or strain will create low back pain that centers primarily over the PSIS (posterior superior iliac spine) with, in more serious cases, pain radiation down the lateral thigh, but above the knee. Pain can sometimes be relieved by sitting and aggravated by walking or repeated bending and twisting.

Objective: All nerve tension signs are negative but there is pain over the PSIS upon palpation. Straight leg raise is normal and there is no increase in pain with sitting, coughing and sneezing as in a lumbar disc syndrome. In moderate to severe cases the joint may "click" or "clunk" during activity if there is hypermobility.

Assessment: Decreased localized pain with increased range of motion.

Laser Treatment Plan: Place the probe over the superior and the inferior part of the joint to deliver 25 to 100 joules per region. Painting over the joint and treatment of tender points in the gluteal region and the lateral thigh may help reduce symptoms. Treat two to three times, over a period of one to two weeks, or until symptoms have significantly decreased. Utilize a maximum of 50–600 joules per session.

Adjunctive Treatment Plan: Mobilization can often provide rapid, short-term relief. Initial use of ice and then later use of ice/heat can be helpful to decrease inflammation and control symptoms. Patient should only perform gentle exercises that provide relief from pain in early stages. Often, active and passive hip flexion and extension exercises can "self-mobilize" the joint and provide relief. In the subacute stage, progress to stabilization exercises and strengthening of core muscles. If one week of treatment has not produced significant improvement, consider referral to an orthopedic specialist.

Spinal Hypermobility Syndrome

(diagram page 67, dose page 66)

Subjective: Patients with hypermobility complain of injury from very mild activity. They easily sprain and strain connective tissues and find that they heal slowly. They often report that their spine "clicks" without provocation.

Objective: There may be "clicking" and "popping" with motion testing and joint play is soft at end-range. Range of motion is normal or excessive, even after an acute sprain. X-rays are usually negative but flexion and extension views can often show increased joint translation.

Assessment: There is pain relief with laser and rest, but no change in the hypermobility. Patients need to be reminded that, if they are careful to avoid serious injury, they will stabilize as they age and their symptoms will lessen. Beighton's Test is a good screening tool.

Laser Treatment Plan: Begin with 10 to 200 joules directly over any area that presents with pain and inflammation with a similar amount of joules painting over the generalized area. Treat with 2–3 times the above dose to achieve a prolotherapy effect.

Adjunctive Treatment Plan: Taping is often beneficial when there is joint instability and more severe cases can benefit from bracing. Patients must be encouraged to do regular gentle strengthening and stabilization exercises and must avoid deep stretching. In some cases prolotherapy (sclerosing) can be beneficial. Consider a referral to an orthopedic specialist if symptoms do not stabilize.

Spine & Pelvis Diagrams

Typical Treatment Time and Joules based on Power of Probe

Probe Output (mW)	Joules	Treatment Time
10	6 - 12	10 - 20 mins
100	36 - 72	6 - 12 mins
500	60 - 180	2 - 6 mins
1,000	90 - 240	1.5 - 4 mins
2,000	120 - 360	1 - 3 mins
3,000	180 - 450	1 - 2.5 mins
4,000	240 - 480	1 - 2 mins
6,000	270 - 570	0.75 - 1.5 mins
10,000	300 - 600	0.5 - 1 mins

The above chart notes the approximate treatment times based on the power of the probe being used. Since the suggested treatment doses in this book are for LEDs and lasers in the range of 10 to 10,000 mW, full body treatment times will be approximately 1–15 minutes and approximately 100 to 1200 joules. If you are using a lower power laser or LED, you will need to use longer treatment times, and proportionally less joules.

Use this chart as a guide for an approximate treatment time and dosage based on your particular laser or LED and the individual needs of the patient.

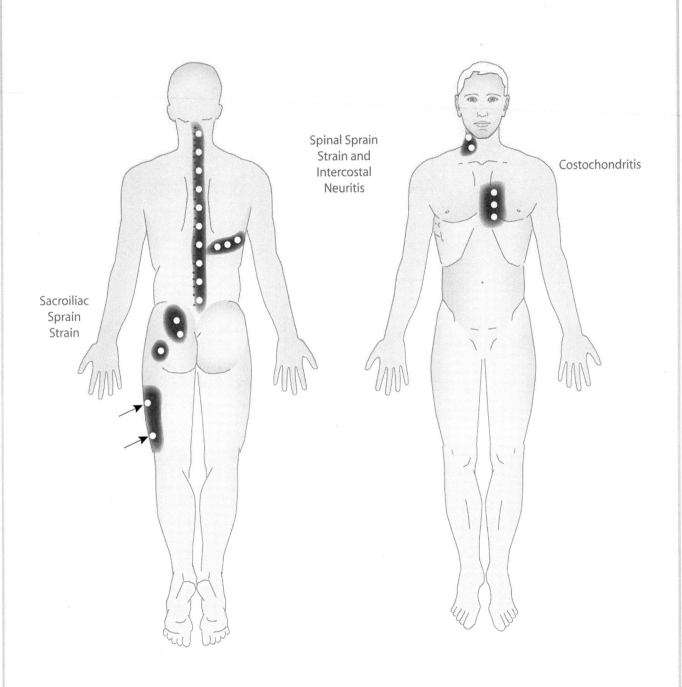

Spinal Sprain
Strain and
Intercostal
Neuritis

Costochondritis

Sacroiliac
Sprain
Strain

Spine & Pelvis

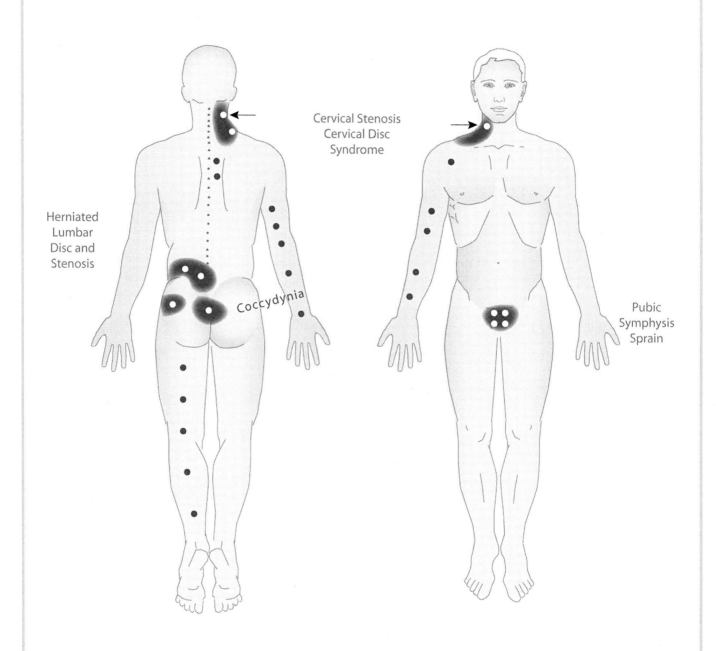

Cervical Stenosis
Cervical Disc
Syndrome

Herniated
Lumbar
Disc and
Stenosis

Coccydynia

Pubic
Symphysis
Sprain

Systemic Treatments

Addiction to Cigarettes or
Other Substances (diagram page 79, dose page 78)

Subjective: This indication is presently experimental, but does show promising anecdotal results. Addiction to almost any substance can be treated, but smoking seems to be especially responsive. Addiction to food and narcotics seems to be more difficult to treat.

Objective: There are numerous tests to substantiate addiction, but these are generally unnecessary.

Assessment: Craving will often be reduced after short-term treatment. Addiction to food and other highly addictive substances can be more difficult and requires other adjunctive treatments.

Laser Treatment Plan: Treating acupoints and ear points with 100 to 300 joules total per session may provide a decrease in cravings. The most effective treatment protocols involve the use of laser auriculotherapy with some peripheral points on the face, arms and legs.

Adjunctive Treatment Plan: It can be helpful to add other therapies such as group therapy, nutritional supplements, meditation, behavior modification, and guided relaxation.

Ankylosing Spondylitis (diagram page 80, dose page 78)

Subjective: The most common early symptom is inflammatory back pain that often starts during the late teens and could be discovered as late as when patients are 40 to 50 years old. In the early stages patients will complain of morning stiffness with fatigue. Fever and weight loss may occur during active periods of the disease and pain is often worse in the early morning and relieved by activity. Insidious and intermittent flare-ups of pain in the sacroiliac joints with periods of remission are common.

Objective: X-rays document sacroiliitis, physical exam notes a loss of lumbar lateral flexion, and lab tests often demonstrate a positive HLA-B27 test.

Assessment: Laser can produce a temporary decrease in symptoms and can help the patient manage inflammation and use less medication.

Laser Treatment Plan: Use a total of 25 to 200 joules during the initial treatments and increase if there is an improvement in symptoms. Treat with 10 to 100 joules on the top of the joint and an equal amount on the lower part of the joint. Because the joint is "C" shaped, it is necessary to treat top and bottom portions of the joint to adequately perfuse it with photons. Painting over the sacroiliac region and the lumbar spine can also produce good results.

Adjunctive Treatment Plan: Exercise often relieves discomfort, so a program of gentle strengthening, stretching, and cardiovascular exercise is vital. Strengthening the back muscles and gentle extension stretching on a ball or foam roller can help limit the progression of the natural kyphosis commonly associated with the disease. Rheumatologic workup may be necessary and the patient may benefit from the use of allopathic or natural anti-inflammatories.

Arthritis (diagram page 81, dose page 78)

See individual syndromes for more specific treatments of different types of arthritis.

Subjective: There will be swelling, stiffness, and pain. Symptoms may be worse in the morning.

Objective: Positive lab tests will confirm the existence of arthritic symptoms. With moderate to severe symptoms, x-rays and other imaging studies will be positive.

Assessment: There will be a decrease in swelling and pain. However, with more severe rheumatoid arthritis, laser will manage symptoms but will not provide a lasting cure.

Laser Treatment Plan: Treat most areas with 5 to 25 joules points per point, with smaller joints receiving a total of 25 to 50 joules and larger joints 50 to 600 joules. Remember to treat all four sides of the joint. To improve depth of penetration, place the laser on one spot without moving it. Osteoarthritis seems to respond better than rheumatoid arthritis.

Hands/Fingers: Treat smaller joints like fingers and toes with less joules than larger joints such as the knee and hip. Measure improvement by decrease in stiffness and swelling, pain-free motion, and measuring grip strength with a pinch gauge or dynamometer.

Wrist: Treat around the circumference of the joint with special attention to the primary area of pain.

Elbow: Identify areas of tenderness, and laser over the lateral and medial epicondyles as well as the adjacent soft tissue.

Shoulder: Causes may be multifactorial, involving the shoulder, acromioclavicular and sternoclavicular joints, muscles, tendons, ligaments, and bursae.

TMJ: Make certain that you treat the TMJ and the adjacent muscles.

Hip: The most efficient access to the acetabulum is best accomplished from the groin (anterior acetabulum) and sciatic notch.

Knee: Soft tissues around the knee, such as the subpatellar and suprapatellar tendon and ligaments, respond more quickly than problems deep within the joint.

Ankle: It is important to treat the area where the problem resides, such as the subtalar or talocrural joint.

Foot/Toes: Smaller joints such as the fingers and toes usually require no more than 25 to 50 joules per joint. With smaller joints and a larger cluster probe, many of the photons are lost because of the poor alignment between the probe and the rounded joint structure.

Adjunctive Treatment Plan: Gentle stretching and range of motion activities are beneficial. Some patients find improvement in symptoms with a combination of oral glucosamine sulfate and MSM (methylsulfonylmethane).

Complex Regional Pain Syndrome or Reflex Sympathetic Dystrophy
(diagram page 82, dose page 78)

Subjective: RSD or CRPS is a very painful syndrome that can cause swelling, redness, temperature changes, and moderate to severe pain. It usually occurs in the hands or feet, although it can occur almost anywhere in the body. The cause of the pain is often due to a minor trauma that surprisingly creates this serious pain condition.

Objective: Initially the only symptom is pain. Later there can be swelling, redness, decreased range of motion, warming or cooling of an area or limb, and even tissue damage that in serious conditions can threaten the viability of a limb. Swelling can result if there is a decrease in the venous and lymphatic circulation, causing an increase of local capillary pressure.

Assessment: There will be a decrease in pain and an associated normalizing of temperature in the symptomatic limb.

Laser Treatment Plan: Treatment can be given two to three times a week for up to three or four weeks to see if laser and light therapy can be of benefit. It is important to start treatment with a very low dose and only increase the dose slowly and carefully, once positive results appear. Positive effects include a decrease in pain and temperature change of one or all of the limbs. Negative effects can be an increase in pain. The first treatment should be no more than 10 to 20 total joules, only increasing if there is no increase in pain.

Start by treating along the transverse processes of the thoracic spine (C7 to L2). This correlates with the sympathetic chain ganglia (SCG). If this does not produce any positive effects, try giving the next treatment to the stellate ganglia (SG), which is located on the anterior lateral transverse process of the seventh cervical vertebra. If symptoms are improved or there is no change, in the next session treat the SCG or the SG with a slightly higher dose, such as 20 to 100 joules. If symptoms are improved or there is no change, in the next session treat the SCG and the SG. If treating the SCG and the SG produces no side effects, try treating the opposite limb and assess if there is any improvement in symptoms. Only treat the symptomatic limb once treatment has been directed to the SCG, SG, and then opposite limb over a series of treatments with no negative side effects or some mild decrease in symptoms.

Adjunctive Treatment Plan: Medical management is imperative and laser therapy must be performed with the approval or supervision of a physician. Range of motion stretching, medication, nutritional counseling, and gentle cardiovascular exercise are vital in maintaining the health of the injured limb.

Fibromyalgia Syndrome (FMS)
(diagram page 83, dose page 78)

Subjective: Most patients complain of morning stiffness and sleep problems. Many complain of feeling as if they have swollen extremities, with numbness and tingling. These symptoms generally are more common in the upper than in the lower extremities.

Objective: The diagnostic criteria for FMS include two basic factors:

1. The presence of pain all over the body for at least three months.

2. The presence of at least 11 of 18 anatomically specific tender points.

The 18 possible tender points exist as nine pairs and may be found at the occiput/nuchal ridge, trapezius, supraspinatus, gluteals, low cervicals, second ribs, lateral epicondyles, greater trochanters, and the medial knees.

Assessment: Improvement is slow and steady.

Laser Treatment Plan: Treat with no more than 25 joules the first treatment, composed of 5 to 10 joules per point. Later, with improving symptoms, dose can be increased to a total full body dose of 50 to 600 joules as long as it is titrated slowly.

Adjunctive Treatment Plan: A multidisciplinary treatment plan composed of exercise combined with education and cognitive behavioral therapy can be highly effective. In addition, gentle manipulation and massage can help decrease stiffness and pain. Daily aerobic and flexibility exercises should be performed at least three times weekly starting gently and slowly increasing in intensity. Warm water aquatic therapy is well tolerated and especially helpful for some patients.

Herpes Zoster/Shingles and Postherpetic Neuralgia

(diagram page 80, dose page 78)

Subjective: Patients complain initially of a small area of painful, red lesions. Over time the severity of pain usually increases and can become severe.

Objective: There will initially be a small area of red, raised lesions. This can increase and eventually spread to a broader area. Herpes most often affects the chest, back, face, and scalp although it may occur almost anywhere. The location of pain or lesions determines the affected dermatome.

Herpes zoster presents in many ways and should be considered a potentially serious problem. It is caused by the Varicella-zoster virus (VZV) and usually warrants an immediate evaluation by a physician. Once VZV infection clears, many individuals continue to suffer pain, called postherpetic neuralgia (PHN). Shingles refers to the painful rash associated with VZV infection and typically affects a single dermatome, most commonly in the thoracic spine. Initially, macules and papules appear and progress to vesicles. The lesions eventually crust and resolve, but many patients experience pain and sensory loss in the distribution of the rash.

Laboratory tests and imaging studies are usually unnecessary.

Assessment: Initially there will be a decrease in pain followed by the disappearance of the lesions.

Laser Treatment Plan: Treatments twice weekly for three weeks is appropriate for acute cases, followed by once per week after there has been a significant decrease in pain. Utilize a maximum of 25 to 100 joules on the first visit.

Adjunctive Treatment Plan: A referral to a physician for anti-viral medication or herbs, laboratory testing, or imaging studies may be necessary in more serious cases.

Postsurgical Pain

Subjective: Pain in the area of the surgery.

Objective: It is common to have redness, swelling, and pain. Make certain that the patient does not have fever higher than 100°F, pain with redness, pus, or swelling at the surgical site, separation of the wound edges, bleeding, shortness of breath, chest pain, a hematoma, vomiting, change in bowel habits, or vomiting. If any of these is present, do not treat and refer immediately to a physician.

Assessment: Pain will be reduced within hours and should create less need for analgesics and anti-inflammatories.

Laser Treatment Plan: First treatment is 25 to 50 joules over the average size wound surface. Raise the dose slowly if there is positive response.

Adjunctive Treatment Plan: Icing the area prior to laser can assist in the reduction of inflammation.

Wounds (Slow or Non-Healing)
(diagram page 80, dose page 78)

Subjective: Patients report impaired healing of wounds. The problem is more common in diabetics and those with circulation difficulties. Make certain that the patient does not have the obvious signs of infection, including fever higher than 100°F, significant pain, increasing redness or faint red lines, heat, chills, lymph swelling or tenderness, pus, or swelling. If there is any suspicion that the wound is infected, refer the patient to a physician immediately.

Objective: Older, non-healing wounds often have a history of infection and may slowly increase in size, provoking fear of the need for surgery or amputation. Other common types of wounds include burns, postsurgical wounds, diabetic ulcers, pressure sores, and venous leg ulcers.

Assessment: The initial goal is to decrease discomfort. The size of the wound will decrease with time as the perimeter begins to heal. Watch for possible signs of infection and refer the patient to a physician if this is suspected.

Laser Treatment Plan: Treatment is ideal after the wound has been cleaned, as the presence of thick, poor-quality tissue will attenuate the absorption of the laser beam.

The most common method is to treat the wound by "painting" back and forth over the wound with a cluster probe. A wound that is 2.5 cm (1 inch) in diameter would need an initial dose of approximately 25 to 100 joules. Treatment can commence daily with decreasing frequency as the wound begins to close and heal. Spend two-thirds of the treatment time on the periphery where there is a higher concentration of actively dividing cells and one-third of the time on the center of the wound where more of the cells are less active. This is done to most effectively stimulate cell growth and improve healing.

If you are using a probe designed to treat acupuncture and trigger points, it is more effective to treat a grid of points that covers the wound. However, it is still important to deliver more of the photons to the periphery than the center of the wound.

Patients may experience an immediate decrease or an increase in pain. Treating with a low dose on the first treatment and then titrating upward with each subsequent session can minimize this reaction.

It is most effective to treat the wound with laser when changing a bandage or dressing. However, it is not imperative to take the bandage off the wound before treating. Using a red or IR cluster probe, it is possible to treat in contact with the sterile dressing. However, you will need to double or triple the dosage because a typical gauze bandage significantly reduces the number of photons passing into the wound.

Wounds can be treated up to two to three times a week, decreasing frequency as the wound heals. It is common for more critical wounds to require 20 visits or more. Less serious wounds can respond after five to ten treatments. Occasional treatments may be necessary afterwards to continue promoting tissue regeneration and complete wound resolution.

Studies show that higher doses are more analgesic and lower doses stimulate healing more effectively. Thus, if healing plateaus before resolution, consider increasing or decreasing the dose to a maximum of 600 joules with a high power probe.

Adjunctive Treatment Plan: Be certain that the wound is not infected by making sure that the physician supervising the treatment is a specialist in wound care. Make sure that the patient has an excellent diet and the wound is cleaned frequently.

Systemic Diagrams

Typical Treatment Time and Joules based on Power of Probe

Probe Output (mW)	Joules	Treatment Time
10	6 - 12	10 - 20 mins
100	36 - 72	6 - 12 mins
500	60 - 180	2 - 6 mins
1,000	90 - 240	1.5 - 4 mins
2,000	120 - 360	1 - 3 mins
3,000	180 - 450	1 - 2.5 mins
4,000	240 - 480	1 - 2 mins
6,000	270 - 540	.75 - 1.5 mins
10,000	300 - 600	.5 - 1 mins

The above chart notes the approximate treatment times based on the power of the probe being used. Since the suggested treatment doses in this book are for LEDs and lasers in the range of 10 to 10,000 mW, full body treatment times will be approximately 1–15 minutes and approximately 100 to 1200 joules. If you are using a lower power laser or LED, you will need to use longer treatment times, and proportionally less joules.

Use this chart as a guide for an approximate treatment time and dosage based on your particular laser or LED and the individual needs of the patient.

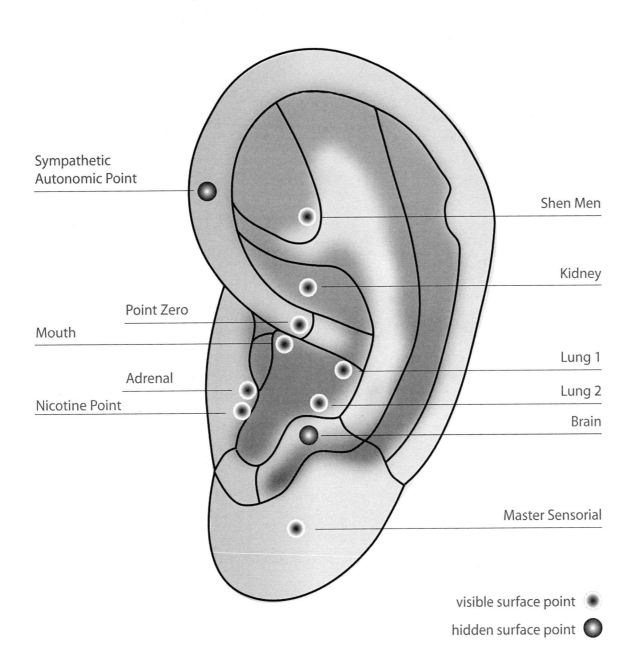

Sympathetic Autonomic Point

Shen Men

Kidney

Point Zero

Mouth

Lung 1

Adrenal

Lung 2

Nicotine Point

Brain

Master Sensorial

visible surface point

hidden surface point

Systemic

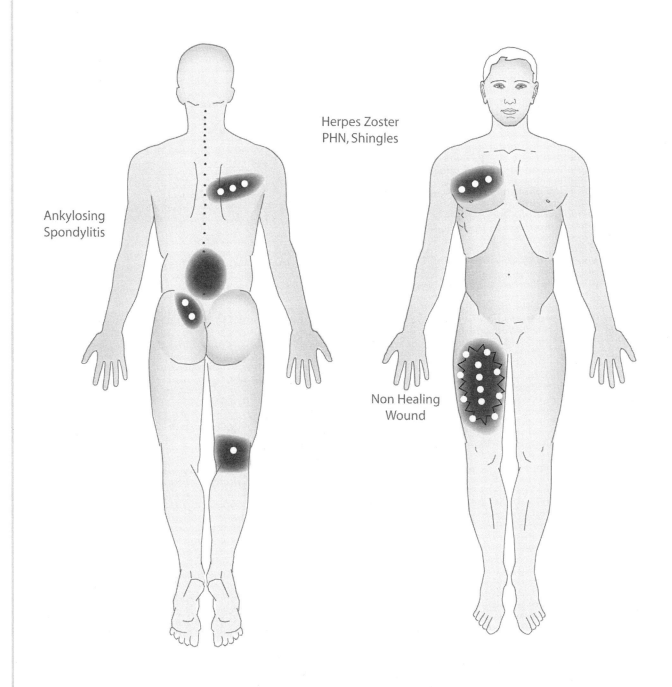

Herpes Zoster
PHN, Shingles

Ankylosing
Spondylitis

Non Healing
Wound

Arthritis

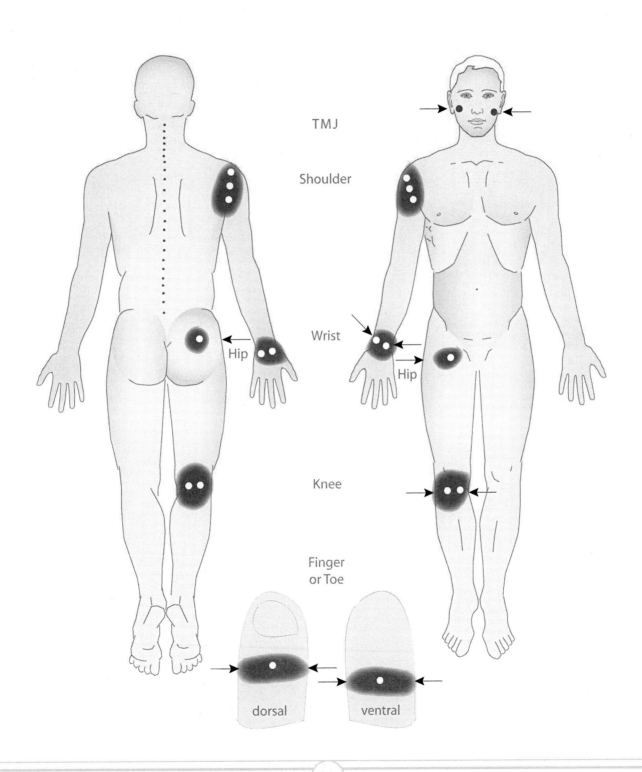

TMJ

Shoulder

Wrist

Hip

Knee

Finger
or Toe

Hip

dorsal

ventral

CRPS

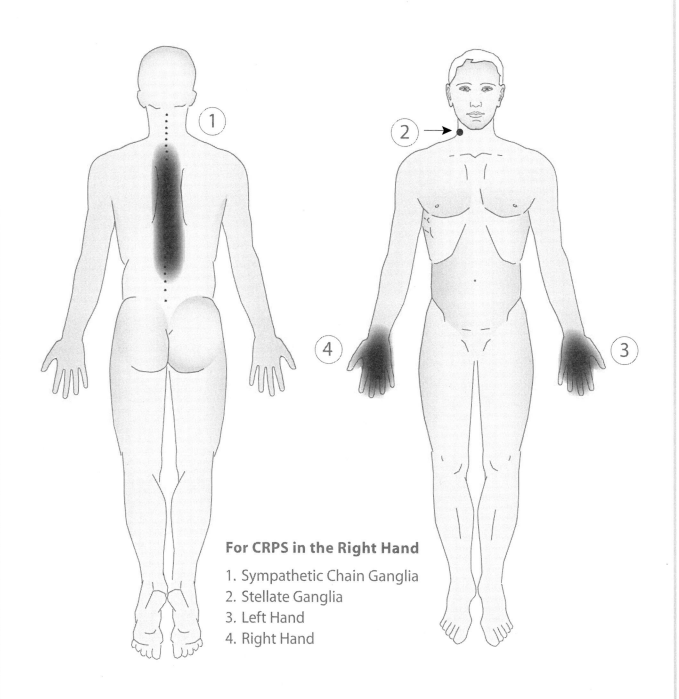

For CRPS in the Right Hand

1. Sympathetic Chain Ganglia
2. Stellate Ganglia
3. Left Hand
4. Right Hand

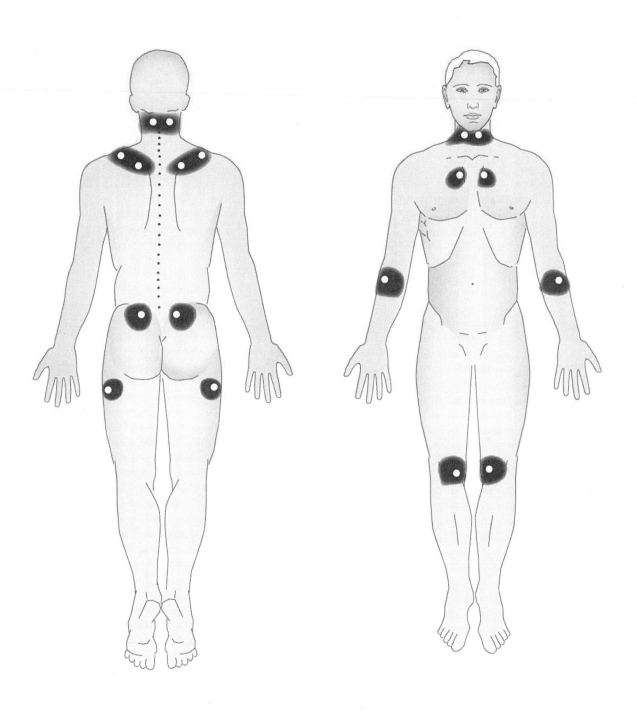

Upper Body Treatments

Acromioclavicular (AC) Sprain or Laxity (diagram page 101, dose page 100)

Subjective: Patients feel pain over the AC joint, and may report "clicking" with motion.

Objective: This injury can result from any blow to the shoulder that disrupts the complex of ligaments holding the clavicle to the acromion process of the scapula. Objective findings are pain on palpation, and when moderate to severe, elevation of clavicle, swelling, and clicking with motion.

Assessment: Improvement results in lessened anatomic clavicle elevation, reduced pain, and increased arm range of motion, especially in abduction.

Laser Treatment Plan: An average treatment dose of 25 to 100 joules is administered at the site, applying 10 to 50 joules to the AC joint followed by painting over the joint and surrounding inflamed tissues. Treatment is focused at the lateral clavicle where it intersects the acromion process. Daily treatments for two to three days can be used during the acute phase followed by treatments one to two times per week. For chronic conditions, use laser prolotherapy with 2–3 times the above dose.

Adjunctive Treatment Plan: Gentle mobilization and exercise, especially arm abductions, are often helpful. If this is difficult, begin by having the patient use their hand to walk up the wall in flexion, later adding abduction. Alternating ice and heat can aid in controlling inflammation and pain. If the joint is unstable, taping may improve stability. If laxity is severe consider referral to an orthopedic specialist for stress x-rays, CT, MRI, bone scan, injections, or surgical intervention.

Biceps Tendinitis (diagram page 101, dose page 100)

Subjective: Patients present with pain on the front of the shoulder/biceps area especially with active and resisted flexion.

Objective: Pain on palpation and on muscle strength testing, swelling and bruising when condition is severe. There can be painfully limited active and sometimes passive range of motion.

Assessment: Improvement will result in reduced pain and swelling, and painless, increased range of motion.

Laser Treatment Plan: With acute conditions use a total dose of 25 to 50 joules, up to a maximum of approximately 600 joules in chronic conditions. This can be administered to the most painful points at the front of the shoulder, with approximately 5 to 25 joules per point. The surrounding area can also be painted with 15–50 joules to reduce swelling and pain. Treat daily for up to three to five days or until symptoms have abated.

Adjunctive Treatment Plan: Taping can help protect the muscle during healing; stretching may be prescribed only after healing of muscle has occurred. Alternating ice and heat may help control inflammation and pain. If the problem persists after appropriate therapy, consider a referral to an orthopedic specialist.

Biceps Tendon Strain (diagram page 101, dose page 100)

Subjective: Pain in the biceps tendon.

Objective: Look for a thin soft spot in the tendon at the point of maximal pain. This is the site of the strain. In moderate to severe tears there can be muscle thickening adjacent to the dented region of the tendon and/or muscle. In more serious cases there will be bruising, with reduced active and normal passive range of motion. Tears occur often from inflammation or weakness in the proximal insertion of the tendon.

Assessment: Pain will decrease and active range of motion will increase.

Laser Treatment Plan: In mild to moderate cases, a total average dose of 25–600 joules can be administered to the attachment points of the tendon plus an equal amount of joules for painting the surrounding area. This may stimulate healing, while reducing bruising, swelling, and pain; it also can be useful in reducing any scarring from surgery. Treat every two or three days until recovery is evident.

Adjunctive Treatment Plan: Prescribe gentle muscle strengthening and stretching once healing has occurred sufficiently to allow the tissues to accept stress. Taping can be used during the acute stage to prevent further tearing and assist in rehabilitation. It can be helpful to alternate ice and heat to control inflammation and pain. If the problem persists after appropriate therapy, consider a referral to an orthopedic specialist.

Carpal Tunnel Syndrome (diagram page 102, dose page 100)

Subjective: Symptoms are numbness and/or pain in the thumb and/or middle three fingers that can increase with activity or at night while sleeping. In moderate to severe cases the pain can be disabling and radiate up into the forearm and arm.

Objective: The symptoms can be reproduced by tapping over the carpal tunnel of the wrist (Tinel's sign). In moderate to severe cases there can be motor loss, positive EMG, and muscle wasting.

Assessment: Successful treatment results produce decreased pain and increased function and strength.

Laser Treatment Plan: The laser must be aimed at the median nerve in the carpal tunnel both vertically and slightly angled to either side of the tendons in the wrist to bathe the entire nerve in photons. A treatment dose of approximately 25 to 100 joules is initially administered in most cases, less if the pain is acute or severe.

It may also be advisable to treat the adjacent tender points in the forearm and hand with 5 to 25 joules per point or perform nerve tracing over the median nerve into the hand. Fingernails can be painted with 10 to 50 joules if additional peripheral stimulation is needed. Always consider the possibility of treating the brachial nerves in the lateral/anterior neck or at the spinal level if you believe that the problem could be cervicogenic.

Treatment can start daily for up to three or four days or until symptoms decrease. Chronic conditions may require higher doses up to 300 joules with a high power laser and frequency can be two or three times a week for up to four weeks.

Adjunctive Treatment Plan: Daily, gentle flexion and extension stretching of the wrist can be added as long as it does not aggravate symptoms. It can be helpful to initially use ice and then alternate ice and heat directly over the carpal tunnel to control inflammation and pain. Many patients find benefit from bracing, especially at night. If the problem persists after appropriate therapy, consider a referral to an orthopedic specialist for injections or surgical intervention.

DeQuervain's Tendinitis
(diagram page 101, dose page 100)

Subjective: Pain at the base of the thumb or lateral wrist.

Objective: Decreased range of motion and, in more chronic cases, thickening of the tendons at the base of the thumb. In performing the Finkelstein test, flexion of the thumb with ulnar wrist deviation will often be painful. X-rays are negative. The disease is an entrapment tendinitis of the tendons of the first dorsal compartment of the wrist.

Assessment: Increasing range of motion and decreased pain.

Laser Treatment Plan: This condition can be treated with approximately 20 to 100 joules. The laser can be administered to tender points along the involved tendon. Treatment can be given two to three times per week for two to six weeks or until relief is obtained. A laser point probe can be helpful.

Adjunctive Treatment Plan: In acute cases ice/heat can assist in symptom control and a splint may be required. In chronic cases, myofascial massage, spray/stretch, home application of ice/heat, thumb flexion stretching, and isometric exercises can be beneficial, when appropriate.

Dislocated Finger or Thumb
(diagram page 104, dose page 100)

Subjective: Severe pain localized to the site of trauma.

Objective: The finger will look deformed due to a dislocation of the carpometacarpal, metacarpophalangeal, or phalangeal articulations. The joint will be swollen and will probably be discolored within one to two days of injury due to spraining of ligaments. The initial stage will probably be treated on the athletic field or in the emergency room.

Assessment: As healing improves there will be increasingly pain-free passive and active range of motion and improved strength.

Laser Treatment Plan: Acute conditions can be treated with a total treatment dose of approximately 25 to 200 joules. Treat at least four points around the joint and follow with painting. For best results, the dislocation should be reduced prior to laser therapy. Treatment can be done daily for three to five days or until the condition is improving rapidly.

Adjunctive Treatment Plan: It can be helpful to initially use ice and then ice/heat to control inflammation and pain. Mobilization or reduction can reduce the dislocation. Start with gentle active range of motion and move to passive and isometric strengthening once the joint is stable. If instability is present, taping can be helpful. If the problem persists after appropriate therapy, consider a referral to an orthopedic specialist.

Fractured Carpal, Metacarpal, or Phalange (diagram page 102, dose page 100)

Subjective: Pain can be mild to severe at the fracture site. The patient may have already been treated by an orthopedic specialist and received x-rays, fracture reduction, casting, and possibly surgery.

Objective: Hairline fractures often present with mild to moderate pain and swelling and can be invisible on x-rays. With moderate to severe injuries, there will be bruising, swelling, and deformity, and they almost always include pain on all ranges of motion and positive findings on x-ray, MRI, CT, or bone scan. Make sure that you look for signs of neurological dysfunction in any wrist injury.

Assessment: Decreased pain and swelling with increased range of motion.

Laser Treatment Plan: Acute conditions can be treated immediately to reduce swelling and pain with about 25 to 200 joules at the site fracture and the surrounding strained soft tissues. If a cast is in place, treatment can be applied to the arteries above the fracture site with 25 to 200 joules per treatment to stimulate healing in the forearm region. You may also treat the radial or ulnar arteries if the cast is on the hand. Once the temporary or plaster cast has been removed, laser treatments may resume two or more times per week until an acceptable level of healing has occurred.

Adjunctive Treatment Plan: In cases of non-union, bone healing may be aided with laser therapy. Be certain that the patient eats a balanced diet and consider multi-mineral supplementation. It can be helpful to alternate ice/heat to stimulate circulation and control inflammation and pain once the cast has been removed. In many cases, there will be decreased range of motion that will require gentle active followed by passive range of motion activities. If the problem persists after appropriate therapy, consider referral to an orthopedic specialist for further evaluation.

Fractured Clavicle (diagram page 103, dose page 100)

Subjective: Mild to severe pain at the fracture site.

Objective: Pain and palpable small elevation of the bone at the fracture site. The fracture is usually visible on x-ray, but some complex cases may require MRI, CT, or bone scan.

Assessment: Decreased pain and swelling indicate improvement.

Laser Treatment Plan: The majority of fractures are in acute or sub-acute conditions and laser can be applied even before x-rays and a sling have been provided to speed healing and reduce swelling and pain. An average treatment dose of 25 to 200 joules is applied directly over and around the fracture site. Treatment can also be initiated soon after diagnosis and treatment by a physician have been completed and the fracture has been stabilized. After the bone has been reset, treatment can be administered every two to three days until pain and swelling have been reduced.

Adjunctive Treatment Plan: In cases of non-union fractures, laser therapy may improve bone healing. Patients should eat a balanced diet and consider multi-mineral supplementation. It can be helpful to initially use ice and later alternate ice/heat to control inflammation and pain. If the problem persists after appropriate therapy, consider a referral back to the orthopedic specialist.

Fractured Distal Radius or Casted Forearm or Hand (diagram page 102, dose page 100)

Subjective: Pain can be mild to severe at the fracture site. The patient may have already been treated by an orthopedic specialist and received x-rays, fracture reduction, casting, and possibly surgery.

Objective: There are numerous fractures of the radius, including the Colles, Galeazzi, Monteggia, and Smiths fractures. There can be bruising, swelling, and deformity of the wrist and almost always pain on all ranges of motion and positive findings on x-ray, MRI, CT, or bone scan.

Assessment: Decreased pain and swelling with improved range of motion.

Laser Treatment Plan: Acute conditions can be treated immediately to reduce swelling and pain, with about 10 to 100 joules at the site of fracture, followed by painting of the surrounding strained soft tissues. Once a cast is in place, treatment can be applied to the arteries above the fracture site, such as the axillary or brachial arteries, starting with 25 to 200 joules per treatment to stimulate healing in the forearm region. You may also treat the radial or ulnar arteries if the cast is on the hand. Once the temporary or plaster cast has been removed, laser treatments may resume to the fracture site, two or more times per week until an acceptable level of healing has occurred.

Adjunctive Treatment Plan: In cases of non-union, bone healing may be aided with laser therapy. Be certain that the patient eats a balanced diet and consider multi-mineral supplementation. It can be helpful to alternate ice/heat to stimulate circulation and control inflammation and pain once the cast has been removed. If the problem persists after appropriate therapy, consider a referral to an orthopedic specialist for further evaluation.

Frozen Shoulder (diagram page 103, dose page 100)

Subjective: Stiffness and pain in and around the shoulder joint, difficulty sleeping, and pain with motion, especially abduction.

Objective: Pain will be felt at the end range of passive or active motion; the joint may be hot and swollen in the rare case of an acute injury. There is usually mild to severe loss of range of motion. Expect pain on palpation at deltoid insertion and along the length of the biceps tendon.

Assessment: Improved active and passive range of motion; lessened pain.

Laser Treatment Plan: Acute conditions can be treated with a total dose of 50 to 600 joules. This can be administered at approximately 10 to 25 joules to various points, directed to the center of the shoulder joint from the anterior, posterior, and superior aspects. The surrounding area may also be painted with approximately 25 to 100 joules. Treatment can be done every two or three days until the patient has achieved 90% of normal range of motion.

Adjunctive Treatment Plan: Passive and active mobilization is a vital part of the therapy. Passive mobilization can be performed in all appropriate directions including posterior, inferior, and lateral glide as well as abduction and adduction. Gentle stretching at home, two to three times per day, is important. It can be helpful to alternate ice and heat to control inflammation and pain. In some cases acupuncture and taping can provide benefit. If the problem persists after appropriate therapy, consider a referral to an orthopedic specialist for manipulation under anesthesia.

Ganglion Cyst of the Wrist

Subjective: Patient complains of a lump near the wrist that may be painful.

Objective: Because ganglions may be caused by a tear of the ligaments between the joints in the wrist, there will be the formation of palpable, fibrous lump.

Assessment: The size and soreness of the cyst will decrease.

Laser Treatment Plan: The treatment of acute ganglions is based on edema reduction of the inflammation in and around the cyst. An average treatment dose of approximately 10 to 100 joules is administered daily for up to three days. The longer the patient has had the ganglion, the less likely it is that there will be significant improvement.

Adjunctive Treatment Plan: Gentle to deep pressure for a few seconds with a laser point probe on top of the ganglion immediately preceding laser treatment may help reduce the size of the cyst. It can be helpful to initially use ice and then alternate ice/ heat to control inflammation and pain.

Olecranon Bursitis (diagram page 101, dose page 100)

Subjective: The patient notices swelling at the posterior elbow that can be painful or painless. There can be a history of trauma or repetitive microtrauma, such as leaning on the elbow repeatedly. Insidious onset does occur.

Objective: This syndrome presents with clearly demarcated, superficial swelling and pain near the olecranon process of the elbow. Range of motion is usually normal or slightly reduced.

Assessment: Decreased pain and swelling with increased range of motion.

Laser Treatment Plan: A total dose of 25–100 joules is applied to the bursae of the olecranon cavity in doses of 10 to 50 joules per point followed by painting over the area near the olecranon process. This can be done two to three times a week until satisfactory relief is obtained.

Adjunctive Treatment Plan: It is recommended that gentle strengthening and stretching be performed once it is no longer extremely painful. It can be helpful to alternate ice and heat to control inflammation and pain. It is recommended to rest the elbow while healing takes place. If the problem persists after appropriate therapy, consider a referral to an orthopedic specialist for an injection or further diagnosis.

Radial or Ulnar Neuritis
(diagram page 103, dose page 100)

Subjective: There can be paraesthesia, muscle contraction, or pain in the forearm or hand, corresponding to the nerve distribution.

Objective: Pain can increase and radiate into the hand with gentle tapping or stretching of the nerve. There is often pain with range of motion of the forearm or hand and it can be accompanied by reflex and motor weakness. X-rays and an EMG can, in some cases, pinpoint a site of entrapment in the neck or upper extremity.

Assessment: Decreased pain with improving strength and pain-free range of motion.

Laser Treatment Plan: The more serious the nerve irritation, the lower should be the initial dose. Start with a total dose of approximately 10 to 25 joules, depending on the severity of symptoms. This can be applied approximately two to three times per week for the first week, decreasing treatment frequency as symptoms improve. Split the treatment time between nerve tracing, the site of entrapment, if it is known, and adjacent tender points.

Adjunctive Treatment Plan: It can be helpful to initially use ice and then alternate ice/heat to control inflammation and pain. If the problem persists after appropriate therapy or there is increasing weakness or muscle spasm, consider a referral to a neurologist or surgeon. As symptoms improve, slowly add gentle stretching and very gentle, simple strengthening exercises.

Rotator Cuff Strain (diagram page 101, dose page 100)

Subjective: Pain is usually felt with abduction. If rupture is moderate or severe, pain can also be present at rest, with swelling, bruising, and muscle weakness.

Objective: Muscle weakness with decreased active range of motion and normal or decreased passive range of motion.

Assessment: Active range of motion will gradually become more pain-free.

Laser Treatment Plan: Acute conditions can be treated with an average dose of 25 to 200 joules applied to the injured area with a combination of point treatment and painting. Treatments should be given every two to three days until satisfactory relief is achieved.

Adjunctive Treatment Plan: Gentle strengthening when there is no pain associated with effort. Taping can help stabilize the muscle during the acute stage. Alternating ice and heat may control inflammation and pain. If the problem persists after appropriate therapy, consider a referral to an orthopedic specialist.

Shoulder Rheumatoid and Osteoarthritis

(diagram page 103, dose page 100)

Subjective: Pain with decreased range of motion and swelling in the shoulder joint.

Objective: Decreased range of motion, swelling, and positive lab tests and/or x-rays.

Assessment: Expect faster results with osteoarthritis than rheumatoid arthritis. Improvement is evident as increased range of motion, with decreased swelling and pain.

Laser Treatment Plan: Acute and chronic arthritis can be treated with a total dose of 25 to 200 joules. This can be directed toward the center of the joint from the superior, anterior, and posterior positions with 10 to 50 joules per point, followed by painting over the entire shoulder region. This will relieve pain in the joint and promote healing. Treat every two to three days for up to three or four weeks until the condition has improved.

Adjunctive Treatment Plan: Gentle range of motion activities can be helpful. Some patients find benefit from glucosamine sulfate and/or MSM. It can be helpful to alternate ice and heat to control inflammation and pain. If the problem persists after appropriate therapy, consider a referral to a rheumatologist.

Subacromial Bursitis (diagram page 102, dose page 100)

Subjective: Pain in the bursa near the impingement site of the deltoid tendon or the head of the humerus where it passes under the acromion process of the scapula.

Objective: Abduction will often produce an impingement sign with pain preventing full range of motion. There may be inflammation, swelling, and point tenderness of the bursa on palpation with pain during abduction. Always check for hypermobility because it can create similar symptoms, without the swollen, tender bursa.

Assessment: Pain will decrease and active range of motion will increase.

Laser Treatment Plan: Acute conditions respond well to laser therapy and will improve rapidly. The total dose is approximately 25 to 200 joules for a mild case. If points are treated, use approximately 5 to 50 joules per point. In the acute stage, treat approximately two to four times per week, decreasing the frequency as symptoms improve. Chronic conditions with other associated shoulder problems can require treatment for up to six to nine weeks.

Adjunctive Treatment Plan: It can be helpful to alternate ice/heat to control inflammation and pain combined with gentle range of motion stretching. In some cases ultrasound, provided after laser therapy, can also be beneficial. Start with flexion stretching and move to abduction as symptoms abate. If the problem persists after appropriate therapy, consider a referral to an orthopedic specialist for an evaluation.

Tennis and Golfer's Elbow

(diagram page 103, dose page 100)

Subjective: This is also called lateral or medial epicondylitis. Pain is present on palpation at the medial or lateral epicondyle tendon attachment sites. Although the problem can occur from participation in sports, almost any repetitive forearm and hand activity can create this condition. Patients may report difficulty lifting a coffee cup or carton of milk, shaking hands, or opening doors.

Objective: There will be pain on palpation near or on the medial and lateral epicondyles. In moderate to severe cases there can be swelling and muscle weakness. In chronic or severe cases MRI will reveal the degree of tearing near or on the attachment site.

Assessment: With increasing healing, there will be less pain, increased ability to lift heavier objects with the hand, and improved functional activities.

Laser Treatment Plan: This condition can be treated with a total average dose of 20 to 100 joules. This dose can be administered to tender points adjacent to the epicondyles as well as directly on the attachment site for 5 to 50 joules per point, followed by painting over the region near the epicondyle. Treatments can be done two to three times a week for two to six weeks, with decreasing frequency as symptoms abate.

Adjunctive Treatment Plan: In acute cases ice and heat can assist in symptom control. In chronic cases, friction, trigger point or myofascial massage, spray/stretch, and gentle strengthening can be beneficial, when appropriate. No massage on the epicondyle is recommended in the acute stage, and stretching should start only after the pain has significantly decreased. Using a tennis elbow brace and taping during upper extremity activitiescan be protective.

Thumb or Finger Sprain

(diagram page 104, dose page 100)

Subjective: Pain with active and/or passive range of motion.

Objective: The severity of a sprain will be proportional to the degree of excessive movement. The joint will be swollen and painful with decreased or increased range of motion. Bruising may follow after the injury. If laxity is severe, refer the patient to an orthopedic specialist immediately.

Assessment: There will be decreasing subjective complaints and improved range of motion and strength.

Laser Treatment Plan: Treatment can be given two to five times the first week and directed into the joint space from all four sides with a total of 25 to 100 joules per session.

Adjunctive Treatment Plan: Gentle active range of motion may be indicated in the first week if it causes no aggravation of symptoms. Passive range of motion or mobilization can be performed once the acute injury has stabilized. It can be helpful to initially use ice and then ice/heat to control inflammation and pain. Bracing and taping can reduce pain and prevent further injury. If the problem persists after appropriate therapy, consider a referral to an orthopedic specialist.

Triceps Strain (diagram page 101, dose page 100)

Subjective: Patients report pain at the site of strain on a portion of the triceps.

Objective: There will be pain on palpation at the primary site of strain and pain on resistive effort when the elbow is straightened. There may be swelling, bruising, palpable tearing, or a "dent" if the strain is moderate to severe.

Assessment: Decreased pain with range of motion and resistive effort.

Laser Treatment Plan: This type of strain can be treated with 5 to 50 joules on each of the most painful points, along with painting over the insertions, body, and origin of the muscle. Treatment can be given daily for up to three days or until the patient feels improved symptoms. The total dose is about 50 to 600 joules per treatment and subsequent sessions can continue twice weekly for up to three to four weeks.

Adjunctive Treatment Plan: Gentle strengthening and stretching, once healing the of the muscle strain has occurred. It can be helpful to alternate ice and heat to control inflammation and pain.

Wrist Flexor or Extensor Tendinitis

(diagram page 104, dose page 100)

Subjective: The patient will notice loss of function due to forearm pain.

Objective: There may be tenderness and inflammation of the tendons of the forearm. Pain will be produced when gripping objects and with any repetitive computer work. There may be a positive jump sign when trigger points are active. In chronic conditions, rigidity and swelling of the tendons are palpable and radiation into the hand, mimicking carpal tunnel syndrome, can occur.

Assessment: Improvement will be noted as decreased pain, increased strength, and improved function.

Laser Treatment Plan: This condition can be treated with a total average treatment dose of approximately 50 to 600 joules. This dose can be administered to tender points, followed by painting. Remember that deeper points require longer treatment times. Treatment can be given once or twice a week for two to six weeks or until relief is obtained.

Adjunctive Treatment Plan: In acute cases initially using ice and then ice/heat can assist in symptom control. In chronic and subacute cases, friction, trigger point or myofascial massage, spray/stretch, home application of ice or heat, and stretching can be beneficial. Night bracing is often protective.

Upper Body Diagrams

Typical Treatment Time and Joules based on Power of Probe

Probe Output (mW)	Joules	Treatment Time
10	6 - 12	10 - 20 mins
100	36 - 72	6 - 12 mins
500	60 - 180	2 - 6 mins
1,000	90 - 240	1.5 - 4 mins
2,000	120 - 360	1 - 3 mins
3,000	180 - 450	1 - 2.5 mins
4,000	240 - 480	1 - 2 mins
6,000	270 - 540	.75 - 1.5 mins
10,000	300 - 600	.5 - 1 mins

The above chart notes the approximate treatment times based on the power of the probe being used. Since the suggested treatment doses in this book are for LEDs and lasers in the range of 10 to 10,000 mW, full body treatment times will be approximately 1–15 minutes and approximately 100 to 1200 joules. If you are using a lower power laser or LED, you will need to use longer treatment times, and proportionally less joules.

Use this chart as a guide for an approximate treatment time and dosage based on your particular laser or LED and the individual needs of the patient.

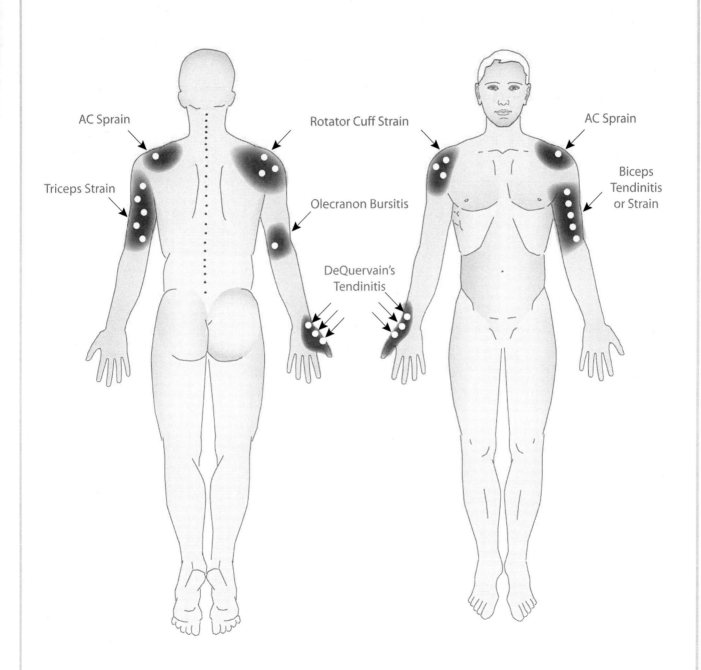

AC Sprain

Rotator Cuff Strain

AC Sprain

Triceps Strain

Olecranon Bursitis

Biceps
Tendinitis
or Strain

DeQuervain's
Tendinitis

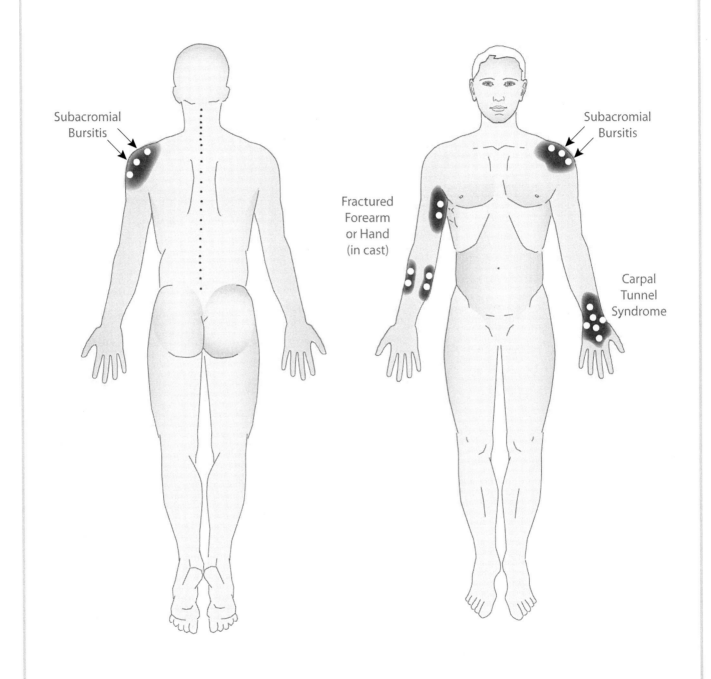

Subacromial Bursitis

Subacromial Bursitis

Fractured Forearm or Hand (in cast)

Carpal Tunnel Syndrome

Upper Body

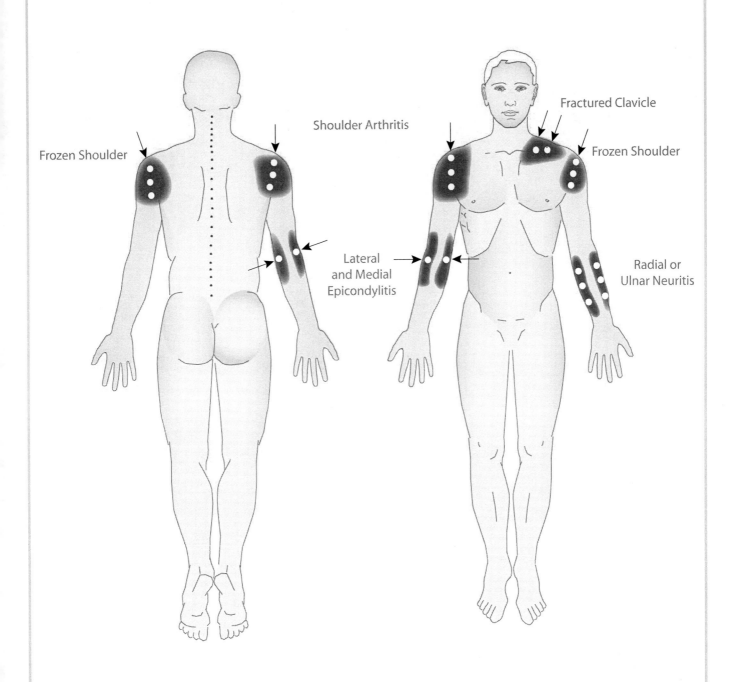

Frozen Shoulder

Shoulder Arthritis

Lateral and Medial Epicondylitis

Fractured Clavicle

Frozen Shoulder

Radial or Ulnar Neuritis

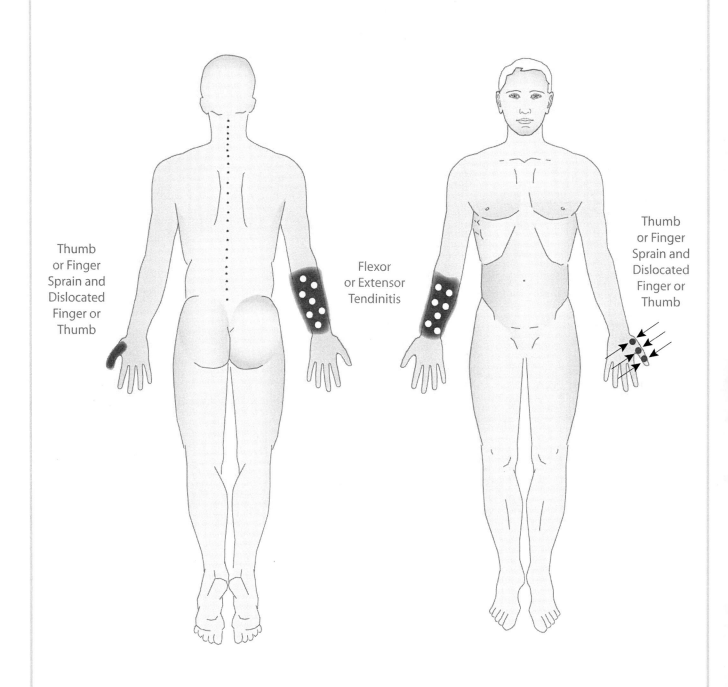

Thumb
or Finger
Sprain and
Dislocated
Finger or
Thumb

Flexor
or Extensor
Tendinitis

Thumb
or Finger
Sprain and
Dislocated
Finger or
Thumb

Lower Body
Treatments

Achilles Tendinitis and Rupture

(diagram page 130, dose page 128)

Subjective: The patient will complain of heel pain or pain in the lower calf. The problem is common in track and field sports, dancers, and not uncommon in the majority of sports.

Objective: There may be a lump within the tendon and pain will be felt when palpating the site of inflammation. In moderate cases a dent will also be felt where the tendon has suffered a partial tear. This I call the "Dent Sign." In severe cases there will be a full tear of the Achilles tendon. If the patient exhibits severe loss of strength in the Achilles, or has a negative Thomas test, an immediate referral to an orthopedic specialist may be indicated.

Assessment: There will be improved ability to do pain-free, standing toe raises.

Laser Treatment Plan: Acute conditions can be treated with a total dose of 50 to 600 joules, with the primary focus being the site of the tendon strain, followed by painting over the general area. Treatment can be given every two to three days, decreasing treatment frequency as the condition heals. Direct the photons from posterior to anterior as well as from a lateral and medial position and at an anterior angle to the tendon to infiltrate its frontal aspect. If the patient has been treated surgically, treat in a similar manner as soon as possible, even daily, until swelling and pain have decreased.

Adjunctive Treatment Plan: When the tendon has healed and the patient can walk pain-free, then gentle stretching of the calf but not the tendon should begin. Wearing heel lifts or high heels can reduce strain on an injured Achilles tendon. Reserve stretching of the tendon and gentle strengthening until the Achilles has fully healed and exercise can be performed without pain. Taping of the tendon can help stabilize the weakened tissue.

Adductor Strain (diagram page 130, dose page 128)

Subjective: Pain near the groin at the adductor attachments that can mimic a sprain of the pubis.

Objective: Palpate for pain and tenderness in the adductor muscles, i.e. adductor longus, adductor brevis, or adductor magnus at the site of their insertion or in the belly of the muscles. There is often pain and weakness with range of motion and strength testing. With severe strains, a "Dent Sign" will be felt near the attachment site where the tendon or fascia has been torn. In chronic conditions the pain can severely limit physical activity.

Assessment: Lessening of pain and increasingly pain-free motion.

Laser Treatment Plan: Treat the attachment site with 10 to 150 joules followed by 10 to 25 joules over any tender points, for a total of 50 to 600 joules per session. Painting over the attachment site with 10 to 50 joules can also be of benefit.

Adjunctive Treatment Plan: Myofascial massage may be performed in the area at least 5 cm (2 inches) distal to injury if it does not provoke or aggravate symptoms. In chronic cases, taping over the attachment to provide stability may help. Suggest active stretching of adductors within a pain-free range of motion once symptoms have stabilized.

Anterior (ACP) and Posterior Compartment Pain (PCP)

(diagram page 130, dose page 128)

Subjective: A patient suffering from ACP will complain of mild to severe pain in the anterior muscles of the lower leg, especially during strenuous exercises such as running up hill or acceleration sports. In severe cases, the pain can become incapacitating. PCP is similar, but creates posterior leg pain and is also aggravated by exercise.

Objective: With PCP there may be swelling and there is pain on palpation on one or more of the following muscles: soleus, gastrocnemius, tibialis posterior, peroneus longus, and the flexor digitorum longus. With ACP there will be pain on palpation on at least one of the following muscles: the tibialis anterior, the peroneus longus, and the peroneus brevis. The fascia over these muscles will feel stiff and may be swollen because the muscles expand more than their fascial sheath and become compressed.

Assessment: Pain and swelling will decrease as the inflammation abates. If the compartment exhibits extreme pain or loss of pulse, refer the patient to an orthopedic specialist immediately.

Laser Treatment Plan: Acute conditions of ACP or PCP can be treated with a total dose of approximately 50 to 600 joules. This can be administered with about 10 to 25 joules per point along each muscle, followed by painting over the entire painful area. This can be done daily for one to five days or until the condition has improved enough to discharge the patient or decrease frequency. Treatment commonly lasts for one to four weeks.

Adjunctive Treatment Plan: Begin self-help, passive stretching of the anterior or posterior compartment. Ice/heat may be used to reduce inflammation and control symptoms.

Anterior and Posterior Cruciate Ligament Injury
(diagram page 132, dose page 128)

Subjective: The patient often complains of a knee "popping," "giving out" or becoming weak. There may be reports of a "click" or a straining sensation in the knee while playing sports that require "cutting" or jumping. The patient may be limping and usually complains that the knee is painful, stiff, and swollen. The severity of the subjective complaints is usually proportional to the degree of ligament strain or rupture.

Objective: There is usually a positive Lachman and Drawer test demonstrating ligamentous laxity, with swelling and decreased range of motion. An x-ray is often inconclusive and an MRI is more likely to accurately assess the degree of ligament damage. If a rupture is suspected, referral to an orthopedic specialist is indicated.

Assessment: Improvement will show as decreased pain and swelling, with improved range of motion. In milder cases, as symptoms improve, there will be less instability with the Lachman and Drawer tests.

Laser Treatment Plan: Acute conditions can be treated with a dose of 25 to 300 joules. Only titrate if improvement is evident with a slow increase in dose. The treatment can be divided into four to five entry points on the knee joint, directed along the joint line, at the posterior, medial and lateral aspects of the knee as well as lateral and medial to the patella. Keep the laser head in one position, if possible, at each point, to increase depth of penetration. Add painting over the knee if pain covers a broad area, or if using a high power laser. Treatment can be given daily for up to five days, followed by decreasing frequency as long as progress is maintained.

Adjunctive Treatment Plan: If the knee cannot be flexed or extended, the condition should be assessed by an orthopedic specialist. Straight leg-raising exercises, with the knee in a gently extended position, and, when pain free, gentle use of the stationary bike, can be used to tone the quadriceps. Begin additional strength training as soon as possible, teaching the patient unloaded, isometric strengthening exercises before progressing to loading and bending the knee. Strength and agility must be attained before the patient can engage in more vigorous activities. Ice/heat, taping or a knee brace can support the injury during the acute stage. Serious ruptures usually need to be surgically repaired.

Calcaneal Bursitis (diagram page 129, dose page 128)

Subjective: Pain in the back of the heel due to trauma, explosive running, overuse, or even wearing shoes that are too small.

Objective: There is pain and a bump on palpation on the two bursae located just superior to the insertion of the Achilles tendon.

Assessment: There will be a progressive decrease in pain.

Laser Treatment Plan: Use 25 to 200 total joules over the bursae, starting with treatment three times per week for one to three weeks. This can be divided into points of 5 to 25 joules followed by painting over the tendon insertion and bursae to stimulate the entire region.

Adjunctive Treatment Plan: Add gentle calf stretching gradually.

Calf Strain (diagram page 131, dose page 128)

Subjective: There is pain in the gastrocnemius or soleus muscles usually brought on by explosive exercise or excessive stretching. The patient, in moderate cases, may exhibit a limp and have difficulty dorsiflexing the ankle due to spasm.

Objective: There will be pain on palpation and often a palpable spasm at the injury site; in more extreme cases, there can be swelling and bruising in the area a few days after the injury. It is important not to confuse this syndrome with an Achilles tendon tear.

Assessment: There will be a return to pain-free range of motion and normal strength in plantar flexion.

Laser Treatment Plan: An acute calf strain can be treated with a treatment dose of approximately 50 to 600 joules. This can be administered to tender points of about 10 to 25 joules over the most painful points, followed by painting over a larger muscle area. Usually this problem is self-limiting and treatment two to three times per week for one to two weeks will be sufficient. If the strain looks severe, be certain that an Achilles tendon tear is not present.

Adjunctive Treatment Plan: Begin self-help passive stretching as soon as it is comfortable. Do not encourage vigorous activity until the muscle has healed well.

Dislocated Patella (diagram page 132, dose page 128)

Subjective: The patient, often a young athletic girl, will complain that her kneecap "popped out of place." It can be caused by a sudden blow or by twisting of the knee. If it is dislocated, refer the patient to an orthopedic specialist. It is not uncommon for the patients to reposition it themselves. The kneecap is swollen and limping may be present due to pain. However, in mild to moderate cases the pain may be minimal.

Objective: Swelling will occur within a few hours after injury. If this swelling causes moderate to severe pain, refer the patient to an orthopedic specialist for an MRI to rule out internal knee damage.

Assessment: Pain-free range of motion will increase as swelling decreases.

Laser Treatment Plan: The majority of these injuries will heal themselves, but often leaves the patient's knee in a more vulnerable state. Use laser prolotherapy 1–2 times per week using 100–500 joules or until the patella is stable.

Adjunctive Treatment Plan: Begin strength training as soon as possible, teaching unloaded and isometric strengthening exercises before progressing to exercises that load and bend the knee. Taping or a knee brace can support the injury during the acute stage.

Hallux Valgus and Rigidus

Subjective: There is often painful motion of the hallux that can cause difficulty walking. Bunions may be associated with arthritis, genetics, or an occupation that involves long term standing and lifting. People with flat feet or those who wear shoes that are too tight, too narrow, or too pointed are more susceptible to bunions.

Objective: Hallux valgus (Bunions) is a lateral deviation and inflexibility of the hallux on the first metatarsal and often includes enlargement of the first metatarsal head.

This presents problems when walking or exercising because it prevents dorsiflexion.

Assessment: With proper treatment there will be a decrease in pain and inflammation. Occasionally, there will be a decrease in lateral deviation of the hallux.

Laser Treatment Plan: Begin with a dose of 25–200 joules, treating two times per week. Direct the laser at the superior, inferior, and medial portion of the first metatarsal head.

Adjunctive Treatment Plan: Often, treatment involves conservative steps that may include orthotics, taping, strapping, and self-help exercises. Severe cases may require surgery to relieve pain and increase function.

Hamstring or Ischiogluteal Bursitis and Tendinitis (diagram page 129, dose page 128)

Subjective: There is tenderness of the proximal or distal insertion of one of the hamstring muscles of the posterior thigh. This can occur with the biceps femoris, semimembranosus, and semitendinosus.

Objective: Palpation will reveal tenderness of the bursae situated underneath the muscle.

Assessment: With improvement there will be decreased tenderness on palpation and increasingly pain-free activity.

Laser Treatment Plan: The hamstring bursa or tendon can be treated with a dose of about 25 to 200 joules. Following this, tender points can be treated or the area can be painted with approximately 10 to 50 joules. The pain is often significantly reduced after two to five treatments in the acute stage, slightly more with chronic conditions.

Adjunctive Treatment Plan: Stretching the hamstring with the leg slightly adducted or abducted, depending on the muscle involved, can improve flexibility in the medial and lateral compartments. Use of ice/heat for five minutes, five times per day can help in the acute stage of injury.

Hamstring Strain (diagram page 130, dose page 128)

Subjective: Pain in the back of the thigh with hip flexion or resistive effort. Pain will be felt over a localized area. There may be localized bruising a day or two after the actual incident of injury, and stretching and touching the area can also elicit pain.

Objective: There will be pain when palpating or stretching the hamstring muscles, with weakness and pain during muscle testing. Injuries to the middle of the muscle belly usually heal faster than those at the proximal attachment site.

Assessment: As the muscles heal there will be less pain with functional activities.

Laser Treatment Plan: Acute conditions can be treated with a total dose of approximately 25 to 100 joules directed over the site of painful points in the muscle followed by painting the surrounding area with approximately 25 to 200 joules. Treatment can be given daily at first, reducing to three times per week until the condition has been healed.

Adjunctive Treatment Plan: Patients should not begin a program of stretching until muscle stretch is pain-free, to limit the likelihood of re-injury.

Hip Sprain (diagram page 130, dose page 128)

Subjective: Pain will be felt in the middle of the groin and may radiate to the thigh or knee. In many ways, this condition may resemble a pubic sprain, groin strain, or hip arthritis. However, unlike with arthritis, there may be an acute incident, involving extreme hip extension or flexion precipitating this injury. Note also that hip arthritis rarely occurs in patients under 50 years old.

Objective: There will be mildly to moderately decreased range of motion with pain felt on end range. Range of motion will be normal, or excessive if there is hypermobility.

Assessment: Treatment will create a rapid decrease in symptoms.

Laser Treatment Plan: Treat with 50 to 600 joules directly over the anterior acetabulum. Posterior treatment of the acetabulum can be accomplished by treating the sciatic notch and aiming the photon stream toward the hip socket. Treatment two times per week for one to two weeks is often sufficient for a mild to moderate injury.

Adjunctive Treatment Plan: Gentle active range of motion can be encouraged but extreme passive or active range of motion should not be performed until the joint has fully healed. Strengthening of the hip muscles is imperative.

Interdigital Neuritis—
Metatarsalgia—
Morton's Neuroma (diagram page 131, dose page 128)

Subjective: Many patients present with an intermittent dull ache, cramping, numbness or burning, and occasional shooting pain in the plantar aspects of the metatarsal interspaces. Symptoms usually worsen with weight-bearing activity and improve with rest.

Objective: In chronic cases a lump of scar tissue will form and there is a palpable mass under the ball of the foot, which will be painful when weight is applied to the metatarsal heads. Pain can also be increased on palpation over the metatarsal heads.

If the toes are hyperextended at the metatarsal joints, the interdigital nerves are tractioned over the transverse metatarsal ligaments. This can cause pressure on the nerves, which can aggravate this syndrome. This condition is most common in the second or the third interspace and in middle-aged persons.

Assessment: With treatment, there will be decreased pain, numbness, and cramping, and improved functional activities.

Laser Treatment Plan: Acute and chronic conditions can be treated with a dose of 50 to 300 joules. This can be directed at the interdigital nerves between the metatarsal heads, especially using a point probe.

Adjunctive Treatment Plan: It can be helpful to alternate ice/heat to control inflammation and pain. Referral to a podiatrist or orthopedic doctor for orthotics, injections, or surgery may also be necessary if there is no improvement.

Knee Contusion, Housemaid's Knee, Prepatellar Bursitis (diagram page 131, dose page 128)

Subjective: The patient complains of swelling, more than pain, which is usually above the tibial tuberosity but can also be superior to the patella.

Objective: This condition produces swelling in the soft tissues that is easily visualized and palpated. In moderate to severe cases there will be difficulty bending the knee.

Assessment: Swelling will decrease slowly and steadily.

Laser Treatment Plan: The area of swelling can be treated with 25 to 200 joules directly over the apex point of swelling followed by painting over the general superior tibial region with another 10 to 100 joules. Treatment can be given daily for up to three to five days, with decreasing frequency until the condition has been healed.

Adjunctive Treatment Plan: If there has been no history of trauma, patients should avoid kneeling and have their feet checked for excessive pronation. If the swelling produces pain, redness, and heat around the tibial tuberosity, suspect infection and refer the patient to a physician.

March or Stress Fracture

(diagram page 132, dose page 128)

Subjective: There will be pain in the midfoot, including the possibility of pain in the navicular, cuboid, or one of the cuneiform bones. There is often a history of repeated running, jumping, etc.

Objective: There will be pain on palpation of the foot and x-rays are often negative.

Assessment: Pain will be lessened and x-rays will be normal.

Laser Treatment Plan: A March fracture can be treated with a total average treatment dose of 50 to 300 joules. This can be delivered to points at approximately 5 to 25 joules, directed over the fracture site. Treatment can be done every two or three days until the condition is fully healed.

Adjunctive Treatment Plan: Be certain that the patient has a good diet and assess the need for mineral supplementation. If the Stress or March fracture was due to a relatively minor physical stressor, a scan would be appropriate to rule out osteoporosis.

Medial and Lateral Collateral Ligament Injury (diagram page 130, dose page 128)

Subjective: The patient will usually complain of pain at the lateral and/or medial joint line. There may be a history of jumping or "cutting" during sports activity, but many cases result from minor twisting movements. Swelling in the area of strain is common.

Objective: Lateral and medial stress testing will show laxity that is proportional to the degree of strain. In mild cases the only symptom will be tenderness along the medial or lateral joint line. In moderate to severe cases, there may be swelling and bruising present. Pain will also be felt when performing medial or lateral stability testing with a valgus or varus stress to the lower leg.

Assessment: There will be less swelling and improved pain-free range of motion with an increased sense of stability and strength.

Laser Treatment Plan: Acute conditions can be treated with a dose of 25 to 200 joules, increasing the dose to a maximum of 600 joules. Only increase the dosage if the condition shows improvement with each small step of titration. This can be directed at the medial and lateral joint line. Keep the laser head in one position at each point, if possible, to increase depth of penetration. Add painting over the medial and lateral region if there is more generalized swelling. Treatment can be done daily for up to three to five days, followed by decreasing frequency as long as progress is maintained.

Adjunctive Treatment Plan: If the knee cannot be flexed or extended, an orthopedic specialist should assess the patient immediately. Institute active, isometric straight leg raising and progress to other isometrics and more aggressive strength training as symptoms improve. Taping can prevent further injury and allow more pain free activity.

Meniscus Sprain/Strain
(diagram page 130, dose page 128)

Subjective: The patient will complain of pain deep inside the knee and often recall an instance of a feeling that something snapped or strained.

Objective: When the medial and/or lateral meniscal cartilage of the knee joint becomes inflamed due to strain or tearing, the knee will swell within the first few hours thereafter and can stay swollen for days to weeks, depending on the severity of the strain. The knee may also feel weak, like it is going to buckle, or lock into one position. An MRI will usually improve the accuracy of this diagnosis. Always test for damage to the anterior and posterior cruciate ligaments as the two syndromes can occur simultaneously.

Assessment: There will be less swelling and increasingly pain-free range of motion with an improved sense of stability and strength.

Laser Treatment Plan: Acute conditions can be treated with a dose of 25 to 100 joules. In some cases up to 600 joules per session will be needed. Only increase the dosage if condition shows improvement with each gentle titration. This can be directed to the medial and lateral joint line, the posterior knee, and points just lateral and medical to the patella. Keep the laser head in one position in each point, if possible, to increase depth of penetration. Add painting all over the knee if swelling is present. Treatment can be given daily for up to five days, decreasing frequency as long as progress is maintained.

Adjunctive Treatment Plan: If the knee cannot be flexed or extended, an orthopedic specialist should assess the patient immediately. Institute straight leg raising exercises with the knee in a gently extended position and do not add knee flexion until it is comfortably tolerated and only in the subacute phase. Taping is important to stabilize the joint. Once the knee is stable, very gentle joint mobilization may improve mobility if there is reduced range of motion.

Metatarsalgia—Thinning of the Fat Pad

(diagram page 131, dose page 128)

Subjective: Pain in the plantar aspect of the foot beneath the metatarsals, increased with impact activities and weight bearing.

Objective: Palpation will reveal a thinning of the fat pad beneath the metatarsophalangeal joints and there will be pain on palpation.

Assessment: Gradual lessening of the pain.

Laser Treatment Plan: Metatarsalgia can be treated with a total dose of 25 to 100 joules. Direct 5 to 50 joules per point over the area of pain and/or bruising. Treatment can be given one to three times a week for up to one to two weeks or until there has been significant decrease in pain.

Adjunctive Treatment Plan: Consider the addition of soft padding to the bottom of the patient's shoes or application of moleskin to the bottom of the foot to reduce compression while standing or walking.

Osgood Schlatter Syndrome

(diagram page 129, dose page 128)

Subjective: The patient complains of pain, especially with physical exertion, on the superior tibia. This problem usually occurs in teenagers due to overloading of the attachment site during vigorous exercise. It can be more common when the child undergoes a growth spurt and can also be aggravated by kneeling or excessive pronation.

Objective: The tibial tuberosity, just below the patella, can be enlarged and is almost always painful to palpation. There is often pain squatting and with resisted knee extension.

Assessment: There will be decreased pain with increasing physical activity as improvement continues.

Laser Treatment Plan: Acute conditions can be treated with a dose of 10 to 100 joules in the initial stage of inflammation. The laser can be placed directly over the tibial tuberosity with 10 to 25 joules, followed by a similar dose to the patella ligament, followed by painting with 10 to 25 joules over the superior tibia. Treatment can be given two times per week until the tibial tuberosity has less pain associated with gentle physical activity.

Adjunctive Treatment Plan: Begin with gentle, passive thigh extension to stretch the quadriceps and consider protective taping. Do not begin aggressive stretching or sports until gentle exercise is pain-free. If the problem persists, refer the patient to an orthopedic specialist for x-rays and a diagnostic workup.

Osteochondritis Dissecans

Subjective: The patient complains of pain, swelling, and tenderness inside the knee that can occur after trauma or a growth spurt in a teenager.

Objective: Pain on palpation and visible swelling. These symptoms plus the feeling of soreness inside the knee are usually due to damage to the blood supply to the condyles and the patellar surface of the femur. In moderate to severe situations, this damage might be the result of a loose body inside the joint, i.e. a piece of bone becoming trapped in the joint space; in such cases there may be locking of the knee. An x-ray can confirm this scenario.

Assessment: Improvement will occur in cases when the bone chip has been removed or the damage has not created a loose body.

Laser Treatment Plan: Begin with a total dose of approximately 25 to 200 joules to speed healing and reduce inflammation whether the bone has been removed or not. Treatment can be given daily for up to two to three days, with decreasing treatment frequency as symptoms subside.

Adjunctive Treatment Plan: Start gentle isometric exercises once patient is comfortable. Begin increasing activity once swelling has decreased and there is normal, pain-free range of motion.

Patellar Tendinitis and Quadriceps Insertion Strain (diagrams pages 129 & 131, dose page 128)

Subjective: This strain involves the quadriceps muscles and often includes the rectus femoris, vastus lateralis, vastus medialis, and the vastus intermedius. This muscle group becomes inflamed at their insertion on the superior or inferior patellar regions. Pain can be felt when the superior or inferior end of the patella is touched, walking up and down stairs, or performing any repeated knee flexion and extension. There may also be redness and swelling in the area.

Objective: Pain on palpation and/or swelling is common. The patellar ligaments and tendons may feel stiff and fibrous in more chronic conditions. If the tear is moderate to severe, there will be a thinning of the tendon/ligament which can be felt on palpation compared to the normal, uninjured side. Often there is limitation in hip extension with the knee flexed.

Assessment: There will be decreasing pain and swelling and increased ability to engage in functional and athletic activities.

Laser Treatment Plan: Treat with 25 to 200 joules directly over the inflamed tendon/ligament, angling the probe posteriorly, medially and laterally to bathe all sides of the knee in photons. Treatment is usually effective when provided one to two times per week; more frequent sessions can be helpful in the most severe cases. Often two to ten treatments are necessary depending on the chronicity of the condition.

Adjunctive Treatment Plan: Hip extension stretching can be helpful, if appropriate, adding strengthening exercises as rehabilitation progresses. It can be helpful to use alternate ice/heat to control inflammation and pain. If the problem persists after appropriate therapy, consider a referral to an orthopedic specialist.

Patellofemoral Syndrome
(diagram page 132, dose page 128)

Subjective: The patient, often an athlete, will complain of pain around and behind the kneecap with kneeling and physical exertion. The patient often reports "clicking" of the patella or a feeling that the kneecap is too loose. This condition is common among teenage females with a tendency toward ligamentous laxity.

Objective: In moderate to severe cases, there will be swelling around the knee and pain behind the patella when the patella is compressed. There may also be clicking sounds at the back of the patella.

Assessment: The patient will report decreasing symptoms with activity and swelling will decrease.

Laser Treatment Plan: A total dose of approximately 25 to 100 joules per session can be administered. Direct the probe to the anterior and posterior patella. Best results may require prolotherapy with a dose of up to 300–600 joules. Treatment can be a applied daily for two to five days or until the pain is alleviated. Begin strength training to muscles that stabilize the patella as soon as it is pain-free.

Adjunctive Treatment Plan: Bracing, taping the patella, and strength training to improve stability can be helpful. In many cases, stretching of the ITB can also be of benefit.

Peripheral Neuropathy (PN)

(diagram page 130, dose page 128)

Subjective: Symptoms may include numbness, loss of balance, burning, tightness, hypersensitivity to touch, and motor weakness in the feet and/or legs.

Objective: There will be numbness and loss of strength as the disease progresses. The causes of PN can be due to heredity, diabetes, the side effects of medication, and toxic exposure. However, in most cases, the onset is insidious. Lab testing to rule out diabetes and other physiologic causes can be of value. Imaging studies and EMG/NCV testing are of limited value but can define severity and rule out other pathologies.

Assessment: A small percentage of patients will achieve complete remission after 4 to 12 sessions, but most will get temporary relief for 1 to 5 days.

Laser Treatment Plan: Start with 10–100 joules per foot and increase dosage if treatment is well tolerated. PN is difficult to treat because some patients become more symptomatic after 25 joules of treatment and others feel relief when they receive more than 500 J per foot, for a total of more than 1,000 J! Spend 2/3 of the time treating the most symptomatic points on the bottom of the foot, followed by painting. Spend 1/3 of the time treating the top of the foot or the popliteal fossa to stimulate the popliteal artery.

Adjunctive Treatment Plan: In general, optimal weight, a regular exercise program, a balanced diet, nutritional supplements, and limiting alcohol consumption can reduce symptoms. Some physicians have found that topical and oral L-Arginine can be of benefit. Nutritional support often involves a multivitamin and mineral formula with Alpha Lipoic Acid, L-carnitine, Benfotiamine, B vitamins, and other nutrients.

Piriformis Syndrome (diagram page 130, dose page 128)

Subjective: Patients will complain of pain in the buttock region. In moderate to severe cases, the pain will radiate into the posterior or lateral thigh, calf or foot, depending on the severity of the impingement. Symptoms can look like sciatica, although there is usually an insidious onset.

Objective: Nerve tension and reflex signs are usually normal as well as lumbar range of motion. Sometimes there is perceptible tightness of the piriformis muscle and deep palparion should reproduce the pain. MRI and CT scan can rule out other pathologies.

Assessment: Improvement results in rapidly lessening of symptoms.

Laser Treatment Plan: Treat the piriformis with 10 to 100 joules followed by 10 to 25 joules over any tender points. Painting over the belly of the muscle and attachment sites with 25 to 200 joules can also be appropriate.

Adjunctive Treatment Plan: Myofascial and trigger point massage can be beneficial. Ice/heat as well as passive and active stretching are vital and can produce a rapid decrease in symptoms.

Plantar Fasciitis (diagram page 129, dose page 128)

Subjective: The typical pain pattern is sharp pain along the middle to posterior arch of the sole of the foot. It may occasionally occur with a heel spur. Patients complain of plantar pain, particularly with the first few steps in the morning or after periods of inactivity. Excessive weight, pregnancy, repeated damage from jumping and other high impact activities, and flat feet can be causative.

Objective: Excessive pronation (eversion) of the foot can result in microtears of the plantar fascia. This excessive stretch of the fascia can result in chronic inflammation of the fascial fibers. If a heel spur is present, x-rays will be positive.

Assessment: Treatment often results in a slow, steady decrease in pain and improved ability to engage in impact activity.

Laser Treatment Plan: Start with 25–100 joules and titrate up slowly if there is an improvement in symptoms after each session. Half of the treatment should be focused on the painful points in the plantar fascia with the other half of the joules utilized painting over the symptomatic area. Begin treating three times per week and decrease frequency as symptoms improve.

Adjunctive Treatment Plan: During the acute phase, the patient should use ice or ice/heat on a regular basis. Taping and orthotics can be helpful. The patient should focus on non-weight bearing activities such as swimming and bicycling. In the subacute phase, regular stretching of the sole of the foot and Achilles can be valuable. As the plantar fascia heals and to reduce scar tissue, massage of the plantar fascia, can be quite helpful. If conservative therapy is not successful, referral to a podiatrist or orthopedic specialist is necessary.

Posterior Knee Swelling—Baker's Cyst

(diagram page 132, dose page 128)

Subjective: The patient will complain of posterior knee swelling. In moderate to severe cases there will be a decrease in knee flexion and mild pain.

Objective: Inspection reveals a lump on the middle, posterior side of the knee and is usually more obvious after exercise. It can accompany an arthritic knee and can wax and wane.

Assessment: Treatment will reduce swelling and improve flexion.

Laser Treatment Plan: A total average treatment of 50 to 600 joules can be administered with the majority of cases, directly applying 10 to 25 joules to the swelling and the remainder provided by painting the surrounding area. Treatment can be given daily for two to three days, decreasing frequency of therapy as condition improves until the pain and swelling has been alleviated.

Adjunctive Treatment Plan: If the lump does not respond to treatment, or is hot and inflamed, an assessment by an orthopedic specialist is indicated.

Quadriceps Strain (diagram page 129, dose page 128)

Subjective: The patient will report pain in the anterior thigh.

Objective: There will be pain on palpation and pain with resistive effort in one of the four quadriceps muscles. In moderate to severe cases there will be a lump in the muscle adjacent to a depression where the muscle or fascia is torn.

Assessment: Increasingly pain-free range of motion and decreased pain with muscle contraction.

Laser Treatment Plan: Acute conditions can be treated with an average dose of approximately 25 to 200 joules directed over the site of tear. Then paint and treat points in the surrounding area with about 10 to 25 joules per point for a total of 100 to 150 joules per session.

Adjunctive Treatment Plan: Gentle active stretching can be done once it is pain-free. Passive stretch cannot begin until there is no pain with activity.

Restless Leg Syndrome or Leg Cramps

(diagram page 129, dose page 128)

Subjective: Patients complain of involuntary sudden movement of the legs. In many cases patients may be unaware of having Restless Leg Syndrome (RLS) until it is brought to their attention when they kick a companion while sleeping. Leg cramps are also usually present.

Objective: There are no objective tests, but the syndrome is easily defined by subjective complaints. There will usually be tender points in the muscles of the lower extremity.

Assessment: Patients will report a decrease of involuntary kicks while sleeping and/or have fewer cramps.

Laser Treatment Plan: Treat trigger, tender or acupuncture points in the low back, hip and lower extremity with 10 to 25 joules per point. Treatment can be applied two times per week for two to three weeks.

Adjunctive Treatment Plan: Regular gentle leg and foreleg/calf stretching is vital. Sometimes stretching after heat can improve the effectiveness of the stretching. Make sure the patient has good nutrition and proper intake of minerals.

Sesamoiditis (diagram page 129, dose page 128)

Subjective: There will be pain and bruising beneath the great toe and sometimes difficulty bending the toe. Often there is a history of impact activities provoking the pain.

Objective: The sesamoid bones will be tender to palpation and dorsiflexion of the toe will increase the intensity the pain. Restricted motion of the first metatarsophalangeal joint (MTP) and/or pain on palpation of a sesamoid bone may also be present. An examination by an orthopedic specialist, including x-rays and/or a bone scan, can confirm the diagnosis.

Assessment: There will be a decrease of pain to palpation beneath the great toe with increasingly pain-free range of motion.

Laser Treatment Plan: Initial treatment should be given two to three times per week with an average treatment dose of 15 to 50 joules. This can be administered to the most painful points with approximately 3 to 5 joules per point followed by painting over the involved area.

Adjunctive Treatment Plan: Sesamoiditis is an overuse syndrome. Some sports performed with cleats can focus excess strain on the first MTP or sesamoid bone and forefoot valgus. A pes cavus structure can be a biomechanical cause. Treatment consists of avoiding stressful weight bearing in the acute phase and limiting dorsiflexion with taping. Later, wearing cushioned-soled shoes, taking NSAIDs, and the combination of rest, ice, compression, and elevation can also be helpful. If these measures are not helpful, referral to a podiatrist or orthopedic specialist is necessary.

Shin Splints (diagram page 131, dose page 128)

Subjective: The patient complains of pain along the medial aspect of the tibialis anterior and, in many cases, along the anterolateral tibia, usually following an increase in jogging or hiking prior to onset of symptoms.

Objective: There will be pain on palpation along the anterolateral tibia as well as the medial tibialis anterior tendons. In some cases, the diffuse nature of the syndrome appears like a mild tibial stress fracture.

Assessment: Pain-free walking and then jogging is a sign of tissue healing.

Laser Treatment Plan: Acute conditions of shin splints can be treated with a total average treatment dose of 25 to 200 joules. This can be administered to tender points with 10 to 25 joules per point followed by painting the surrounding area.

Adjunctive Treatment Plan: Make sure that the patient has good lower extremity biomechanics and good athletic shoes. Begin gentle strength training to the anterior compartment muscles as soon as it is comfortable and add stretching and massage once the tissue is in the subacute stage.

Sprained Ankle (diagram page 131, dose page 128)

Subjective: Ankle pain with stiffness.

Objective: Decreased ankle range of motion with swelling and occasionally bruising on the lateral ankle due to ligament damage following forced inversion. If a fracture is suspected, an x-ray should be performed.

Assessment: There will be increased range of motion, less pain and decreased swelling.

Laser Treatment Plan: A sprained ankle can be treated with a total average dose of 50 to 300 joules. This can be administered to the local area of the sprain with approximately 5 to 15 joules per point, especially on the lateral aspect, followed by painting over the whole ankle. Treatment can be given every two to three days for one to three weeks or until the condition is healed.

Adjunctive Treatment Plan: A strength and conditioning program can be helpful. Encourage the patient to warm up before practice or competition and use tape to stabilize the ankle. It may be important to use an ankle brace and supportive shoes in some cases. If the condition becomes chronic or the patient is a competitive athlete, use of a balance board and other ankle exercises to increase strength, balance, and proprioception may be indicated.

Tarsal Tunnel Syndrome

(diagram page 132, dose page 128)

Subjective: The patient may complain of sharp pain, numbness, and muscle weakness on the medial ankle and foot.

Objective: Tarsal tunnel syndrome is a condition in which the posterior tibial nerve is trapped in its tunnel underneath the talocalcaneal ligament. A Tinel's test applied just posterior to the medial malleolus can trigger symptoms.

Assessment: Pain and numbness will be reduced, muscle strength will increase, and Tinel's sign will be negative.

Laser Treatment Plan: Acute and chronic conditions can be treated with a total treatment dose of 25 to 200 joules focused on the posterior tibial nerve. Place most of the photons into the site of impingement, which is usually on the anterior aspect of the medial ankle, and then trace the nerve along the medial foot, and into the lateral plantar aspect of the foot.

Adjunctive Treatment Plan: It can be helpful to alternate ice and heat to control inflammation and pain. Podiatric or orthopedic treatments, including orthotics, injections or surgery, may also be necessary if there is no improvement in symptoms. Check for flat feet; for some patients, the medial stress of flat feet can aggravate this condition and, in such cases, recommend the use of plantar arch supports.

Tensor Fascia Lata and Iliotibial Band Syndrome (diagram page 130, dose page 128)

Subjective: The patient complains of pain above or below the greater trochanter. It may present as a point of pain or mimic sciatica and radiate from the lateral buttock into the lateral knee. This is a common problem in runners and other athletes, but can also be associated with an earlier bout of sciatica or in out-of-shape patients who do not engage in regular stretching.

Objective: Palpation will reveal local tenderness in the tensor fascia lata (TFL) muscle and/or in the iliotibial band (ITB) and can continue down the thigh, where the muscle attaches to the lateral condyle of the tibia. There may be point tenderness with palpation of the lateral femoral condyle or lateral tibial condyle, especially when flexing or extending the knee and over the greater trochanter. Tightness of the ITB may be noted upon examination with an Ober or Thomas test.

Assessment: Treatment should result in less pain on palpation, increased flexibility, improved range of motion, and a return to pain-free activity.

Laser Treatment Plan: Acute conditions can be treated with a dose of 25 to 50 joules. In some cases, if the patient tolerates the treatment well, increasing to 100–300 joules may be indicated if both conditions are present. Treatment can be administered above and below the greater trochanter and distally to the lateral condyle of the tibia. Treat each tender point with 5 to 25 joules and then paint over the entire symptomatic area.
Adjunctive Treatment Plan: When treating athletes, it may be important to encourage them to have a coach assess their athletic form or have a foot specialist watch their gait

and lower extremity biomechanics. Myofascial or trigger point massage, self-massage with a foam roll, and spray/stretch may be added to reduce spasm and fibrous adhesions. It can be helpful to institute active stretching of abductors, within a pain-free range, once the patient's symptoms have stabilized. Reduce activity to a level that does not generate pain and try applying ice/heat to the region of pain along the ITB or TFL to control symptoms.

Tibial or Fibula Stress Fracture

(diagram page 131, dose page 128)

Subjective: The patient complains of pain along the shaft of the tibia or fibula.

Objective: Pain to palpation will be felt on the bone at the site of the fracture. Sometimes one can perceive a slight depression in the bone or even swelling at the primary trauma site. In most cases a bone scan or x-ray will confirm the diagnosis.

Assessment: There will be pain-free walking, running, and stretching.

Laser Treatment Plan: Acute conditions can be treated with approximately 25 to 200 joules. This can be administered at about 25–50 joules per point along the painful aspect of the tibia or fibula. Treatment can be given every one to two days until improvement is evident.

Adjunctive Treatment Plan: Often gentle weight bearing and later strength training will help stimulate healing. Avoiding anything that aggravates the pain is very important.

Trochanteric Bursitis (diagram page 129, dose page 128)

Subjective: This syndrome provokes complaints of pain around the greater trochanter that may radiate down the thigh and mimic sciatica. It is common in runners and in patients who do not stretch their hip abductors. Trochanteric bursitis is caused by painful inflammation of the bursa that is superficial to the greater trochanter. Patients typically complain of lateral hip pain that may radiate down the lateral aspect of the thigh and into the knee.

Objective: Palpation reveals acute pain and possibly swelling of the bursa in an area over or adjacent to the greater trochanter. Typically, symptoms worsen when the patient is lying on the affected bursa or exercising.

Assessment: With improvement there will be decreased pain when walking, exercising, and on palpation.

Laser Treatment Plan: Treat two to three times the first week, decreasing therapy frequency as symptoms improve. Use 25 to 200 joules directly over the bursa followed by painting over the general area with 25 to 200 joules.

Adjunctive Treatment Plan: It is often beneficial to apply a few minutes of gentle trigger point pressure with your hands or a T-Bar directly over the inflamed bursa. This can be followed or preceded by laser therapy. Use of ice/heat for five minutes, five times per day can help in the acute stage of injury. It is important that the patient engages in stretching the iliotibial band (ITB) and tensor fascia lata (TFL). In some cases self-massage and use of a foam roller may also be of benefit.

Lower Body
Diagrams

Typical Treatment Time and Joules based on Power of Probe

Probe Output (mW)	Joules	Treatment Time
10	6 - 12	10 - 20 mins
100	36 - 72	6 - 12 mins
500	60 - 180	2 - 6 mins
1,000	90 - 240	1.5 - 4 mins
2,000	120 - 360	1 - 3 mins
3,000	180 - 450	1 - 2.5 mins
4,000	240 - 480	1 - 2 mins
6,000	270 - 540	.75 - 1.5 mins
10,000	300 - 600	.5 - 1 mins

The above chart notes the approximate treatment times based on the power of the probe being used. Since the suggested treatment doses in this book are for LEDs and lasers in the range of 10 to 10,000 mW, full body treatment times will be approximately 1–15 minutes and approximately 100 to 1200 joules. If you are using a lower power laser or LED, you will need to use longer treatment times, and proportionally less joules.

Use this chart as a guide for an approximate treatment time and dosage based on your particular laser or LED and the individual needs of the patient.

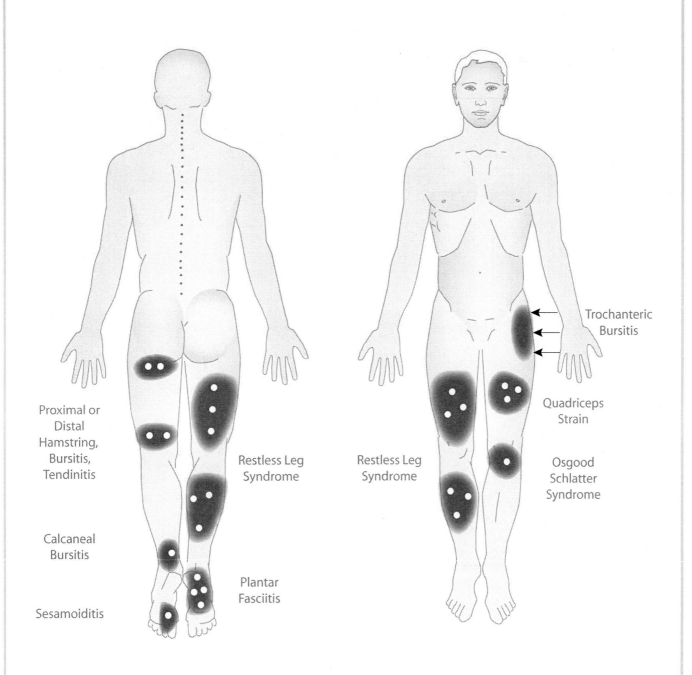

Proximal or
Distal
Hamstring,
Bursitis,
Tendinitis

Restless Leg
Syndrome

Calcaneal
Bursitis

Plantar
Fasciitis

Sesamoiditis

Restless Leg
Syndrome

Trochanteric
Bursitis

Quadriceps
Strain

Osgood
Schlatter
Syndrome

Lower Body

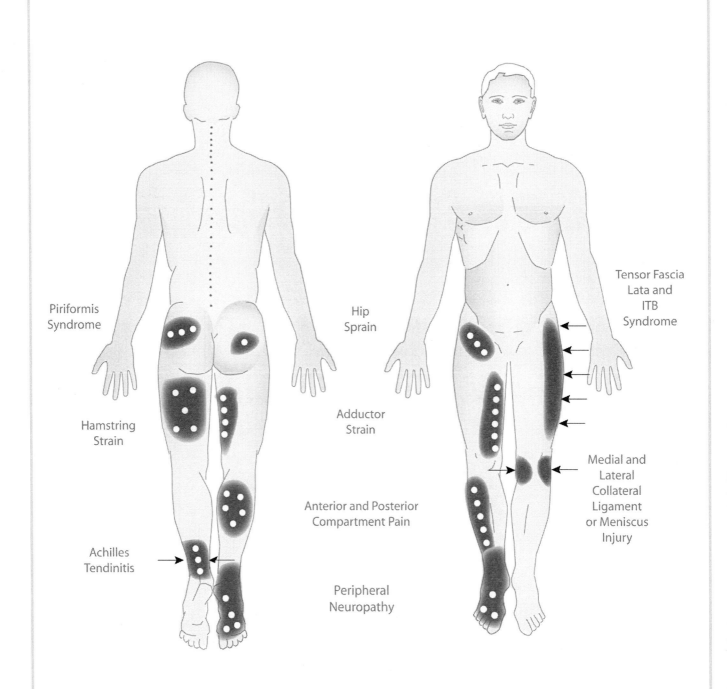

Piriformis
Syndrome

Hamstring
Strain

Achilles
Tendinitis

Hip
Sprain

Adductor
Strain

Anterior and Posterior
Compartment Pain

Peripheral
Neuropathy

Tensor Fascia
Lata and
ITB
Syndrome

Medial and
Lateral
Collateral
Ligament
or Meniscus
Injury

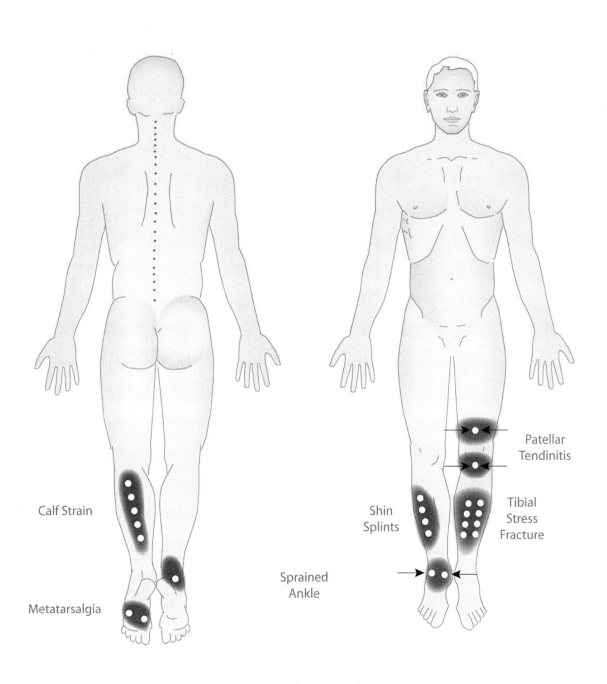

Calf Strain

Metatarsalgia

Shin
Splints

Sprained
Ankle

Patellar
Tendinitis

Tibial
Stress
Fracture

Lower Body

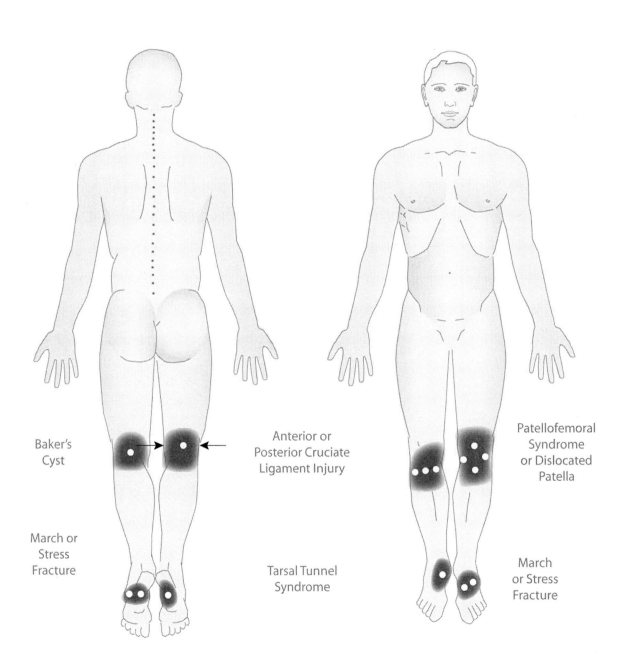

Baker's Cyst

Anterior or Posterior Cruciate Ligament Injury

Patellofemoral Syndrome or Dislocated Patella

March or Stress Fracture

Tarsal Tunnel Syndrome

March or Stress Fracture

Brain
Treatments

Treating the Brain (diagram page 139)

One of the most exciting discoveries in light and laser science has been proof that light can improve healing of the brain. Even though studies began in 2005 on animals and many have been performed more recently on humans, the FDA has not looked at these treatments sufficiently to warrant FDA clearance. However, the compelling data from this research warrants inclusion into any book on light or laser therapy. I will present some basic protocols for treating the brain based on the latest research. If you are interested in learning more, there are many excellent studies coming out of the Wellman Centers for Photomedicine at Harvard Medical School and Massachusetts General Hospital, as well as many studies from Europe, Asia, and the Middle East.

Be careful

Please exercise caution, as this information is taken from the research literature and is not an **FDA cleared indication for using LEDs or lasers.** We legally cannot treat the brain. However, remember that whenever you treat the head for headaches or muscular head pain (like the temporalis muscle), you are also treating the brain! The same thing occurs when you treat over the spine for back pain. You are, in fact, treating the spinal cord as well!

Benefits have been proven

We are not sure exactly how light and laser therapy improves brain function, but we do know that it has many positive effects that can last for weeks or months after treatment. These long-term changes must be due to a significant improvement with brain physiology and function. Some researchers believe it is due to improved ATP synthesis, increased blood flow, or improved oxygenation, even though these probably do not explain all of the long-term improvements that have been noted.

Wavelength

As mentioned in other parts of this book, we do know that there are some wavelengths that are more effective than others. We know that 660 nm and 810 nm are often considered the most effective wavelengths for many types of light and laser therapy because these wavelengths are powerfully absorbed. In general, 810 nm produces the most effective penetration and is the most thoroughly studied. Studies show that higher wavelenths produce very deep penetration as well. These longer wavelengths above 1,000 nm can be effective, but because they generate more heat, especially with higher power lasers, they tend to be avoided in brain research.

LED vs. Laser

We are now seeing an increase in the use of LEDs rather than lasers in brain research and for other types of light and laser therapy because they are less expensive and quite effective. This may make them more useful than lasers when treating the brain, unless the laser has a low total output power and power density, to ensure that it is cool and safe. For example, a high-powered 10,000 mW hot laser has risks when treating the brain that do not occur with a lower power laser or an LED. Lastly, because the world is moving toward the use of LEDs instead of incandescent light bulbs for home and commercial lighting, the quality, durability, power, and price of LEDs is becoming more attractive.

Dosage

Dosage is a controversial subject when treating spine and extremity injuries, but it becomes more complex when treating the brain. In summary, it has been shown that, in the human skull, penetration could reach approximately 1–2 inches (40–50 mm). Whether you are treating animals or humans, it has also been shown that earlier intervention and repeated treatments are the most effective way to produce long-lasting results. From what we see in the literature, one treatment to an area of old brain trauma will be unlikely to produce any significant benefit.

Here is a typical treatment protocol:

Let's invent a study that uses a 500 mW LED that is applied to each side of the forehead for 4 minutes. If you have a 3,000 mW probe, you would reduce the time proportionally:

1. So, 4 minutes (240 seconds) divided by 6 equals 40 seconds. Because a 3,000 mW probe is 6 times stronger than a 500 mW probe, you would reduce the dose to 1/6 of the dose compared to a lower power light device.

2. Thus, you could gently paint over each side of the prefrontal cortex for 40 seconds.

3. However, if we assume that your 3,000 mW probe is an 810 nm laser and the study used an 830 nm LED, which is less intense, you probably want to reduce the treatment to 20–30 seconds on each side of the forehead because lasers are a more intense light than an LED.

4. Note: Since a 3,000 mW probe produces 180 joules per minute and you treat both sides of the forehead for 30 seconds, your total dose would be about 180 joules. However, remember that only a small percentage of those joules reach the brain!

Where Do You Treat?

Most of the studies treating emotional and cognitive function treat the prefrontal cortex. However, a study of Parkinson's disease applied light to the brain stem, as well as the occipital, parietal, temporal, and frontal lobes, and along the sagittal suture. Treating the sagittal suture, because it is just superior to the saggital sinus, could be an excellent area of treatment to improve blood and CSF flow. Remember that studies show that light has systemic effects, so you can treat almost anywhere in the body, even the feet, and have a mild effect on the brain!

If you are interested in learning how the researchers decidced what areas to treat, just do an Internet search on "Brain Function Map" and you will find lots of resources to help guide your studies.

Brain Treatment Diagram

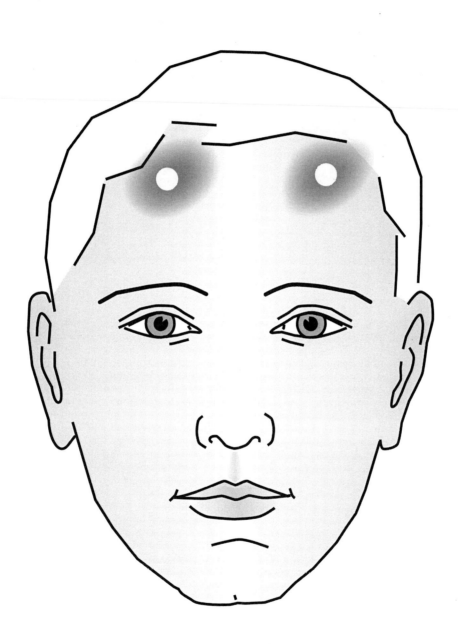

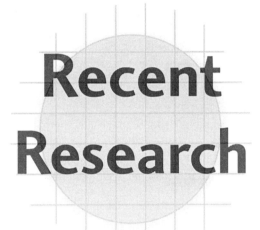

Recent Research

AUTONOMIC NERVOUS SYSTEM BENEFITS
Irradiation of the Stellate Ganglion reduced VAS scores and increased local temp due to an increase regional blood flow by a reduction in vascular tone
Hashimoto et al., Laser Therapy 1997 (9) pp 7–12.

AUTONOMIC NERVOUS SYSTEM BENEFITS
LLLT improves ANS function
Lasers Surg Med. 2014 Dec;46(10):796–803.

BACTERIA AND VIRUSES
LLLT can inhibit some bacteria and viruses.
Lett Appl Microbiol. 2016 Mar;62(3):230–6.
Lasers Med Sci. 2016 Apr;31(3):549–56.
Antiviral Res. 2014 Oct;110:70-6.

BONE REGENERATION
Laser improves osteoblastic formation, bone strength in fractures, implant stability, and can improve osteonecrosis of the jaw.
Lasers Med Sci. 2010 Jul;25(4):559–69).
J Orthop Surg Res. 2010 Jan 4;5(1):1.
J Photochem Photobiol B. 2016 Oct;163:14–21.

CARDIAC PATHOLOGY BENEFITS
LLLT improves cardiac function.
Photomed Laser Surg. 2016 Nov;34(11):516–524
Lasers Med Sci. 2016 Nov 17.

CARPAL TUNNEL SYNDROME
Meta-analysis demonstrated that low-level laser improved hand grip, pain, and sensory nerve function.
Medicine (Baltimore).2016 Aug;95(31): 4424.

CELL AND PHYSIOLOGICAL BENEFITS
INCREASES: Cell proliferation, cell division, cell maturation, secretion of growth factors, wound healing, collagen production, wound strength, wound closer, fibroblasts, myofibroblasts, chondrocytes, epithelialization, skin circulation, oxygen supply, activity satellite cell cultures (stem cells).
DECREASES: Prostaglandin E2, substance P, cyclooxygenase 2 (Cox 2), muscle tension.
J Clin Las Med Surg 2004; 22 (2)141–150.

CELLULAR BENEFITS
INCREASES: Mitochondria and ATP production, Cytochrome oxidase and singlet oxygen, tissue regeneration genes and motor proteins, RNA DNA synthesis, growth factors, cell metabolism, angiogenesis, and mitosis.
Desmet K, et al. Photomed Laser Surg. 2006 Jun;24(2):121–128.

CORTISONE HAS SIMILAR EFFECTS AS LASER
Animal study; 810-nm laser was almost as good as cortisone at reducing swelling. Higher doses showed most benefit.
Laser therapy reduced joint swelling and correlated with decreased serum prostaglandins.
Castano AP, Lasers Surg Med 2007 Jul;39(6):543–50.

CORTISONE IMPROVED WITH LLLT
Laser plus cortisone more effective than cortisone by itself.
Photomed Laser Surg. 2010 Oct;28(5):639–46.

DEPTH OF PENETRATION
LLLT passing through the skull with an 808 nm wavelength laser penetrated approximately 40 mm (1.6 inches).
Lasers Surg Med. 2015 Apr;47(4):312–22.

808 nm laser produced 1 mW/cm2 was achieved at 3.4 cm (1.36 inches), but for 980 nm achieved only 2.2 cm (less than 1 inch). It was determined that 808 nm of light penetrates as much as 54% deeper than 980 nm light.
Photomed Laser Surg. 2013 Apr;31(4):163–8.

FROZEN SHOULDER BENEFITS
A significant improvement in laser therapy compared to the control group.
The treatment group experienced significantly less pain and significantly improved disability scores. Range of motion in the treatment group was better than placebo.
Photomed Laser Surg. 2008 Mar 16.

HAIR LOSS
Meta-analysis of studies covered in this review found an overall improvement in hair regrowth, thickness, and patient satisfaction following LLLT.
Lasers Surg Med. 2016 Apr 25.

HIGHER DOSES INHIBIT
Lower Doses Stimulate, Higher Doses Inhibit. Using 14X the dose inhibited tissue repair.
J Biophotonics. 2016 Mar 15.

HIGHER DOSES INHIBIT
Lower Doses Stimulate, Higher Doses Inhibit
Cumulative effect of lower doses (2.5 or 5 J/cm(2)) determines the stimulatory effect, while multiple exposures at higher doses (16 J/cm(2)) result in an inhibitory effect with more damage.
Photomed Laser Surg. 2006 Dec;24(6):705–14.

INCREASE MOUTH OPENING, DECREASED MUSCULAR PAIN, DECREASED EATING DIFFICULTY, AND DECREASED TENDER POINTS
Photomed Laser Surg. 2006; 25 (5): 637–80.

INFLAMMATORY MEDIATOR INHIBITION
DECREASES: Inflammatory mediators, Cytokine receptors, Inflammatory proteins, Genes that code for inflammation, Proapoptotic proteins.
Desmet K, et al. Photomed Laser Surg. 2006 Jun;24(2):121–128.

INTENSITY OF THE LASER RADIATION WAS REDUCED BY 66% AFTER BEING TRANSMITTED THROUGH THE SKIN. Most laser radiation was absorbed within the first 1mm of skin.
Acupunct Eletrother Res., 2007;321 (1–2);81-6.

LASER vs. ULTRASOUND AND BRACING
Laser therapy was the only treatment that increased grip strength.
Journal of Hand Therapy, Jan–March 2008

LLLT BRAIN DISORDERS
Harvard research shows that LLLT is a promising treatment for many types of brain disorders.
BBA Clin. 2016 Oct 1;6:113–124.

LOWER POWER DENSITIES SHOWED BEST COLLAGEN STRUCTURE
The best organization of collagen were shown by the lower densities.
All wavelengths and fluences used in this study were efficient at accelerating the healing process, with lower densities better than higher, hotter densities.
Photomed Laser Surg. 2006 Dec;24(6):754–8.

LOW-LEVEL LASER THERAPY VS LOW-INTENSITY PULSED ULTRASOUND (LIPUS)
LIPUS enhanced bone repair by promoting bone resorption; LLLT accelerated this process through bone formation.
Photomed Laser Surg. 2006 Dec;24(6):735–40.

MEDICATION STRONGER WITH LASER
Laser Helps TB Treatment: Laser plus medication better than medication alone for tuberculosis.
Indian J Tuberc. 2010 Apr;57(2):80–6.

MITOCHONDRAL FUNCTION IMPROVED
Improves oxygen production, promoting cellular survival, Increased Cytochrome c oxidase—terminal enzyme of the electron transport chain and a strong photoacceptor and other mitochondral enzymes.
J Photochem Photobiol B. 2006 Nov 17.

MUSCLE PERFORMANCE AND LASER
Meta-analysis of 533 studies showed can increase in muscle mass after training, and a decrease in inflammation and oxidative stress in muscle biopsies.
J Biophotonics. 2016 Nov 22.

NECK PAIN BENEFITS
LLLT improves chronic neck pain and function.
Open Orthop J. 2013 Sep 20;7:396–419.

NERVE GROWTH STIMULATION
Controlled trial showed regeneration of sciatic nerve and myelination in rats.
Rochkind. Photomed & Laser Surg. 2007, 25(3): 137–143.

NERVE HEALING
LLLT accelerates peripheral nerve regeneration.
Lasers Med Sci. 2015 Dec;30(9):2319–24.

NON-STEROIDALS: COMPARATIVE EFFECT
LLLT reduces inflammation and improves function, in some cases superior to NSAIDs.
J Lasers Med Sci. 2016 Winter;7(1):45–50.

ORAL MUCOSITIS
LLLT reduces pain in chemotherapy induced oral mucositis.
J Lasers Med Sci. 2016 Winter;7(1):45–50.

PARKINSON'S IMPROVED WITH LASER
LLL improves nerve function with Parkinson's.
Molecular Degen 2009 Jun 17;4:26

PENETRATION UP TO 23 CM
Lasers and LED's of Optimal Wavelength Penetrate up to 23 cm (4 studies).
Desmet K, et al. Photomed Laser Surg. 2006 Jun;24(2):121–128.

PERIPHERAL NEUROPATHY
LLLT helps patients with diabetic peripheral neuropathy.
Acta Med Iran. 2013 Sep 9;51(8):543–7.

PHYSIOLOGICAL BENEFITS
INCREASES: cell proliferation, cell division, cell maturation, secretion of growth factors, wound healing, collagen production, wound strength, wound closer, fibroblasts, myofibroblasts, chondrocytes, epithelialization, skin circulation, oxygen supply, activity satellite cell cultures (stem cells).
DECREASES: Prostaglandin E2, substance P, cyclooxygenase 2 (Cox 2), muscle tension.
J Clin Las Med Surg 2004; 22 (2)141–150.

PSYCHIATRIC DISORDERS IMPROVED
LLL applied to skull decreased depression and anxiety.
Behavioral and Brain Functions, 2009, 5:46, 8 December 2009.

6% OF PHOTONS REACH SPINAL CORD
Applied directly to SP of porcine subjects; 6% of photons reached cord and increased CGRP/mRNA.
Kimberly Byrnes, PhD, NAALT, 2003/2004.

STROKE
Animal Study; Neurological deficits improved.
Lasers Surg Med. 2006 Jan;38(1):70–3.
Stroke. 2006 Oct;37(10):2620–4.

STROKE HELPED WITH LASER
Laser applied to skull improves brain following stroke.
Curr Cardiol Rep. 2010 Jan;12(1):29–33

TEMPORMANDIBULAR JOINT (TMJ)
Decrease of pain and anti-inflammatory effects; confirmed by thermographic examination.
Photomed Laser Surg. 2006 Aug;24(4):522–7.

TENDINITIS AND MYOFASCIAL PAIN BENEFITS
Acute tendinitis had the best response.
Logdberg-Anersson et al., Laser Therapy 1997 (9) pp 79–86.

TENDINITIS BENEFITS
LLLT proven to help tendinitis.
Acta Ortop Bras. 2015 Jan-Feb;23(1):47–9.

THYROID FUNCTION IMPROVES
Laser improves the function of the thyroid based on lab values with chronic autoimmune thyroiditis.
Lasers Surg Med. 2010 Aug;42(6):589–96.

TOENAIL FUNGUS LASER AT HIGHER TEMPERATURES KILLS FUNGAL SPORES
J Am Podiatr Med Assoc. 2010 May–Jun;100(3):166–77.
Photochem and Photobiol 2009 Nov–Dec;85(6):1364–74.

TRIGEMINAL NEURALGIA BENEFITS
Trigeminal, like most pain syndromes, can benefit from LLLT.
Lasers Surg Med. 2014 Dec;46(10):796–803.

ULTRASOUND vs. LASER
Animal Study; Laser treatment provided a much greater increase in the wound strength than ultrasound.
J Rehab Res & Dev, Volume 41 Number 5, September/October 2004.

Bibliography

Abergel RP, Lyons RF, Castel JC, Dwyer RM, and Uitto J. (1987): Biostimulation of wound healing by lasers: Experimental approaches in animal models and in fibroblast cultures. Journal of Dermatological and Surgical Oncology, 13(2):127–133.

Ad N and Oron U. (2001): Impact of low energy laser irradiation on infarct size in the rat following myocardial infarction. Inter. J. Cardiol, 80:109–116.

Aimbire F, Albertini R, de Magalhães R G, Lopes-Martins R A et al. Effect of LLLT Ga-Al-As (685 nm) on LPS-induced inflammation of the airway and lung in the rat. Lasers in Medical Science. 2005; 20 (1): 11–20.

Aimbire F, Albertini R, Leonardo P, Castro Faria Neto HC, Iversen V V, Lopes-Martins R A B, Bjordal J M. Low level laser therapy induces dose-dependent reduction of TNF-alpha levels in acute inflammation. Photomed Laser Surg. 2006; 24 (1): 33–37.

Akai M, Usuba M, Maeshima T, Shirasaki Y, Yasuika S. (1997): Laser's effect on bone and cartilage: Change induced by joint immobilization in an experimental animal model. Lasers Surg Med, 21:480–484.

Allendorf JDF, Bessler M, Huang J, Kayton ML, Laird D, Nowygrod R, and Treat MR (1997): Helium-neon laser irradiation at fluences of 1, 2 and 4 J/cm2 failed to accelerate wound healing as assessed by both wound contracture rate and tensile strength. Lasers in Surgery and Medicine, 20:340–345.

Al-Watban FAH, Zhang XY (1997): Comparison of wound healing process using argon and krypton lasers. J Clin Laser Med Surg, 15:209–215.

Al-Watban F A, Zhang X Y. The comparison of effects between pulsed and CW lasers on wound healing. J Clin Laser Med Surg. 2004; 22 (1):15–18.

Amat A, Rigau J, Nicolau R, Aalders M et al. Effect of red and near-infrared laser light on adenosine triphosphate (ATP) in the luciferine-luciferase reaction. Journal of Photochemistry and Photobiology A: Chemistry. 2004; 168 (1–2): 59–65.

Anders J J, Geuna S, Rochkind S. Phototherapy promotes regeneration and functional recovery of injured peripheral nerve. Neurol Res. 2004; 26 (2): 233–239.

Bagis S, Comelekoglu U, Coskun B, Milcan A et al. No effect of GA-AS (904 nm) laser irradiation on the intact skin of the injured rat sciatic nerve. Lasers in Medical Science. 2003; 18 (2): 83–88.

Bakhtiary A H, Rashidy-Pour A. Ultrasound and laser therapy in the treatment of carpal tunnel syndrome. Aust J Physiother. 2004; 50: 147–151.

Barberis, G., Gamron, S., Acevedo, G., et al. (1996): In vitro synthesis of prostaglandin E2 by synovial tissue after helium-neon laser radiation in rheumatoid arthritis. J. Clin. Laser Med. Surg, 14:4:175–177.

Barushka O, Yaakobi T and Oron U. (1995): Effect of laser (He-Ne) irradiation on the process of bone repair in the rat tibia. Bone, 16:47–55.

Basford JR. (1993): Laser therapy: scientific basis and clinical role. Lasers Ortho Surg, 16(5):541–547.

Baxter DG. (1999): Therapeutic Lasers Theory and Practice. United Kingdom. Harcourt Publishers, Ltd.

Baxter GD, Bell AJ, Allen JM, Ravey J. (1991): Low level laser therapy: current clinical practice in Northern Ireland. Physiotherapy, 77:171–178.

Bayat M, Delbari A, Almaseyeh M A et al. Low-level laser therapy improves early healing of medial collateral ligament injuries in rats. Photomed Laser Surg. 2005; 23 (6): 556–560.

Bayat M, Vasheghani M M, Razavi N et al. Effect of low-level laser therapy on the healing of second-degree burns in rats: a histological and microbiological study. J Photochem Photobiol B. 2005; 78 (2): 171–177.

Bellamy, N., Bradley, L.A. (1996): Workshop on chronic pain, pain control and patient outcomes in rheumatoid arthritis and osteoarthritis. Arthritis Rheum, 3:357–362.

Bibikova A, Belkin A and Oron U. (1994): Enhancement of angiogenesis in regenerating gastrocnemius muscle of the toad (Bufo viridis) by low energy laser irradiation. Anat. Embryol, 190:597–602.

Bibikova A and Oron U. (1993): Promotion of muscle regeneration following cold injury to the toad (Bufo viridis) gastrocnemius muscle by low energy laser irradiation. Anat. Rec, 235:374–380.

Bibikova A and Oron U. (1994): Attenuation of muscle regeneration in amphibians by low energy laser irradiation. Lasers Surg. Med, 4:355–362.

Bibikova A and Oron U. (1995): Regeneration in denervated toad gastrocnemius muscle and promotion of the process by low energy laser irradiation. Anat. Rec, 241:123–128.

Bjordal J M, Johnson M I, Iversen V, Aimbire F, Lopes-Martins R A. Photoradiation in acute pain: a systematic review of possible mechanisms of action and clinical effects in randomized placebo-controlled trials. Photomed Laser Surg. 2006; 24 (2): 158–168.

Bjordal J M, Lopes-Martins R A, Iversen V V. A randomised, placebo controlled trial of low level laser therapy for activated Achilles tendinitis with microdialysis measurement of peritendinous prostaglandin E2 concentrations. Br J Sports Med. 2006; 40 (1): 76–80.

Bjordal J M. Can a Cochrane review in controversial areas be biased? A sensitivity analysis based on the protocol of a systematic Cochrane review Low Level Laser Therapy in Osteoarthritis. Photomed Laser Surg. 2005; 23 (5): 453–458.

Bouma MG, Buurman WA, and van den Wildenberg FAJM. (1996): Low energy laser irradiation fails to modulate the inflammatory function of human monocytes and endothelial cells. Lasers in Surgery and Medicine, 19:207–215.

Branco K, Naeser MA. (1999): Carpal tunnel syndrome: Clinical outcome after low-level laser acupuncture, microamps transcutaneous electrical nerve stimulation, and other alternative therapies—An open protocol study. Journal of Alternative and Complementary Medicine, 5:5–26.

Broadley C, Broadley KN, Disimone G, Reinisch L, and Davidson JM. (1995): Low-energy helium-neon laser irradiation and the tensile strength of incisional wounds in the rat. Wound Repair and Regen, 3:512–517.

Bromm B, Chen AC. (1995): Brain electrical source analysis of laser evoked potentials in response to painful trigeminal nerve stimulation. Electroenceph Clin Neurophysiol, 95(1):14–26.

Byrnes K R, Barna L, Chenault V M et al. Photobiomodulation improves cutaneous wound healing in an animal model of type II diabetes. Photomed Laser Surg. 2004; 22 (4): 281–290.

Byrnes K R, Waynant R W, Ilev I K Wu X et al. Light promotes regeneration and functional recovery and alters the immune response after spinal cord injury. Lasers Surg Med. 2005; 36 (3): 171–185.

Byrnes K R, Wu X, Waynant R W, Ilev I K, Anders J J. Low power laser irradiation alters gene expression of olfactory ensheathing cells in vitro. Lasers Surg Med. 2005; 37 (2): 161–117.

Cambier DC, Vanderstraeten GG, and Mussen MJ, van der Spank JT. (1996): Low-power laser and healing of burns: a preliminary assay. Plastic and Reconstructive Surgery, 97:555–558.

Ceccherelli F, Altafino L, Lo Castro G, et al. (1989): Diode laser in cervical myofascial pain: a double-blind study versus placebo. Clin J Pain, 5(4):301–304.

Cheng R. (1990): Combined treatments of electrotherapy plus soft laser therapy has synergistic effect in pain relief and disease healing. Surgical and Medical Lasers, 3 (3): 135.

Chow R T, Barnsley L. Systematic review of the literature of low-level laser therapy (LLLT) in the management of neck pain. Lasers Surg Med. 2005; 37 (1): 46–52.

Chow RT, Heller GZ, Barnsley L. The effect of 300mW, 830nm laser on chronic neck pain: A double-blind, randomized, placebo-controlled study. Pain. 2006 Sep;124(1-2):201–10.

Cohen N, Lubart R, Rubinstein S, Breitbart H (1998): Light irradiation of mouse spermatozoa: Stimulation of in vitro fertilization and calcium signals. J Photochem and Photobiol 68: 407–413.

Conlan MJ, Rapley JW, Cobb CM. (1996): Biostimulation of wound healing by low-energy laser irradiation. A review. J Clin Periodont, 23:492–496.

Conlan MJ, Rapley JW, and Cobb CM. (1996): Biostimulation of wound healing by low-energy laser irradiation. Journal of Clinical Periodontology, 23:392–296.

Cowen D, et al. (1997): Low energy helium neon laser in the prevention of oral mucositis in patients undergoing bone marrow transplant: results of a double blind randomized trial. Int J Radiat Oncol Bioi Phys, 38 (4): 697–703.

Crespi R, Covani U, Margarone JE, Andreana S. (1997): Periodontal tissue regeneration in beagle dogs after laser therapy. Lasers Surg Med, 21:395–402.

de Medeiros JS, Vieira GF, Nishimura PY. Laser application effects on the bite strength of the masseter muscle, as an orofacial pain treatment. Photomed Laser Surg. 2005; 23 (4): 373–376.

Devor M. (1990): What's in a beam for pain therapy? Pain, 43:139.

Dyson M, and Young S. (1986): Effect of laser therapy on wound contraction and cellularity in mice. Lasers in Medical Science, 1:125–130.

Ebneshahidi N S, Heshmatipour M, Moghaddami A, Eghtesadi A P. The effects of laser acupuncture on chronic tension headache—a randomised controlled trial. Acupuncture in Medicine. 2005; 23 (1): 13-18.

Eckerdal A, Lehmann B H. (1996): Can low reactive-level laser therapy be used in the treatment of neurogenic facial pain? A double-blind, placebo controlled investigation of patients with trigeminal neuralgia. Laser Therapy, 8:247–252.

El Sayed SO, Dyson M. (1990): Comparison of the effect of multiwavelength light produced by a cluster of semiconductor diodes and of each individual diode on mast cell number and degranulation in intact and injured skin. Lasers Surg Med, 10:559–568.

El Sayed SO, Dyson M. (1996): Effect of laser pulse repetition rate and pulse duration on mast cell number and degranulation. Lasers Surg Med, 19:433–437.

Enwemeka CS. (1988): Laser biostimulation of healing wounds: specific effects and mechanism on action. J. Orthop Sports Phys Ther, 9:333–338.

Enwemeka CS. (1990): Laser Photostimulation. Clinical Management, 10:24–29.

Enwemeka CS. (1992): Ultrastructural morphometry of Membrane-bound intracytoplasmic collagen fibrils in tendon fibroblasts exposed to He:Ne laser beam. Tissue & Cell 24:511–523.

Enwemeka CS, Cohen E, Duswalt EP, Weber DM. (1995): The Biomechanical effects of Ga-As Laser photostimulation on tendon healing. Laser Therapy, 6:181–188.

Enwemeka CS, Rodriguez O, Gall NG, Walsh NE. (1990): Morphometric of collagen fibril population in He:Ne laser photostimulated tendons. J Clin Laser Med Surg, 8:151–156.

Fahey TJ, Sadaty A, Jones WG, Barber A, Smoller B, Shires GT. (1991): Diabetes impairs the late inflammatory response to wound healing. J Surg Res, 50:308–313.

Fargas-Babjak A. (2001): Acupuncture, transcutaneous electrical nerve stimulation, and laser therapy in chronic pain. Clin J Pain, 17(4 Suppl):S105–13.

Fillipin L I, Mauriz J L, Vedovelli K, Moreira A J, Zettler C G, Lech O, Marroni N P, Gonzalez-Gallego J. Low-level laser therapy (LLLT) prevents oxidative stress and reduces fibrosis in rat traumatized Achilles tendon. Lasers Surg Med. 2005; 37 (4): 293–300.

Friedmann H, Lubart R, Laulicht I (1991): A possible explanation of laser-induced stimulation. J Photochem and Photobiol B Biol 11: 87–95.

Ghamsari SM, Taguchi K, Abe N, Acorda JA, Sato M, Yamada H. (1997): Evaluation of low level laser therapy on primary healing of experimentally induced full thickness teat wounds in dairy cattle. Vet Surg, 26:114–120.

Gigo-Benato D, Geuna S, de Castro Rodrigues A, Tos P et al. Low-power laser bio-stimulation enhances nerve repair after end-to-side neurorrhaphy: a double-blind randomized study in the rat median nerve model. Lasers in Medical Science, 2004; 19 (1): 57–65.

Gottlieb T, Jörgensen B, Rohde E, Müller G, Schellera EE. The influence of irradiation with low-level diode laser on the proteoglycan content in arthrotically changed cartilage in rabbits. Medical Laser Application. 2006; 21 (1): 53–59.

Graham DJ, Alexander JJ. (1990): The effects of argon laser on bovine aortic endothelial and smooth muscle cell proliferation and collagen production. Curr Surg, 47:27–30.

Grossman N, Schneid N, Reuveni H, Halevy S, Lubart R. (1998): 780 nm low power diode laser irradiation stimulates proliferation of keratinocyte cultures: involvement of reactive oxygen species. Lasers Surg Med, 22:212–218.

Gruber W, Eber E, Malle-Scheid D, Pfleger A et al. Laser acupuncture in children and adolescents with exercise induced asthma. Thorax. 2002; 57 (3): 222–225.

Gür A, Cosut A, Sarac A J et al. Effect of different therapy regimes of low power laser in painful osteoarthritis of the knee: A double-blind and placebo-controlled trial. Lasers in Surgery and Medicine. 2003; 33: 330–338.

Gür A, Karakoc M, Cevik R et al. Efficacy of low power laser therapy and exercise on pain and functions in chronic low back pain. Lasers in Surgery and Medicine. 2003; 32 (3): 233–238.

Gür A, Sarac A J, Cevik R, Altindag O, Sarac S. Efficacy of 904 nm gallium arsenide low level laser therapy in the management of chronic myofascial pain in the neck: a double-blind and randomized-controlled trial. Lasers in Surgery and Medicine. 2004; 35 (3):229–235.

Gür A,Cosut A, Sarac A et al. Efficacy of different therapy regimes of low-power laser in painful osteoarthritis of the knee: a double-blind and randomized-controlled trial. Laser Surg Med. 2003; 33: 330–338.

Haas AF, Isseroff R, Wheeland RG, Rood PA, and Graves PJ. (1990): Low-energy helium-neon laser irradiation increases the motility of cultured human keratinocytes. The Journal of Investigative Dermatology, 94:822–826.

Haker E, et al. (1991): Is low-energy laser treatment effective in lateral epicondylalgia? J of Pain and Symptom Management, 6(4): 241–246.

Hawkins DH, Abrahamse H. The role of laser fluence in cell viability, proliferation, and membrane integrity of wounded human skin fibroblasts following helium-neon laser irradiation. Lasers Surg Med. 2006; 38 (1): 74–83.

Houghton PE, Keefer KA, and Krummel TM. (1994): Transforming Growth Factor Beta (TGF1) plays a role in conversion of 'scarless' fetal wound healing to healing with scar formation. Wound Repair and Regeneration, 3(1):54–61.

Houghton PE, Keefer KA, and Krummel TM. (1996): A simple method for the assessment of the relative amount of scar formation in wounded fetal mouse limbs. Wound Repair and Regeneration, 4:489–495.

Ihsan F R. Low-level laser therapy accelerates collateral circulation and enhances microcirculation. Photomed Laser Surg. 2005; 23 (3): 289–294.

Iijima K, Shimoyama N, Shimoyama M, Yamamoto T, Shimizu T, and Mizuguchi T (1989): Effect of repeated irradiation of low-power He-Ne laser in pain relief from postherpetic neuralgia. Clin J Pain, 5: 271–274.

Karu T. (1998): The Science of Low-Power Laser Therapy. The Netherlands. Gordon and Beach Science Publishers, (OPA) Overseas Publishers Association.

Kasai S, Kono T, Yamamoto Y, Kotani H, Sakamoto T, and Mito M. (1996): Effect of low-power laser irradiation on impulse conduction in anesthetized rabbits. J Clin Laser Med Surg, 14: 107–109.

Kemmotsu 0, Sato K, Furumido H, Harada K, Takigawa C, Kaseno S, Yokota S, Hanaoka Y and Yamamura T. (1991): Efficacy of low reactive-level laser therapy for pain attenuation of postherpetic neuralgia. Laser Therapy, 3: 71–76.

Khadra M, Kassem N, Haanaes H R, Ellingsen J E, Lyngstadaas S P. Enhancement of bone formation in rat calvarial bone defects using low-level laser therapy. Oral Surg Oral Med Oral Pathol Oral Endod. 2004; 97: 693–700.

Khullar S M, et al. (1996): Low level laser treatment improves longstanding sensory aberrations in the inferior alveolar nerve following surgical trauma. J Oral Maxillofac Surg, 54: 2–7.

Laakso E L, Cabot P J. Nociceptive scores and endorphin-containing cells reduced by low-level laser therapy (LLLT) in inflamed paws of Wistar rat. Photomed Laser Surg. 2005; 23 (1): 32–35.

Lanzafame R J, Stadler I, Coleman J, Haerum B, Oskoui P, Whittaker M, Zhang R Y. Temperature-controlled 830-nm low-level laser therapy of experimental pressure ulcers. Photomed Laser Surg. 2004; 22 (6): 483–488.

Lim HM, Lew KK, Tay DK. (1995): A clinical investigation of the efficacy of low level laser therapy in reducing orthodontic postadjustment pain. Am J Orthod Dentofacial Orthop, 108(6):614–22.

Loegdberg-Andersson M, et al. (1997): Low level laser therapy (LLLT) of tendonitis and myofascial pains—a randomized, double-blind, controlled study. Laser Therapy, 2 (9): 79–86.

Lonauer G. (1986): Controlled double-blind study on the efficacy of He-Ne laser beam versus He-Ne plus infra-red laser beams in the therapy of activated osteoarthritis of finger joints. Laser Surg Med, 6:172.

Longo L, Evangelista S, Tinacci G, Sesti AG. (1987): Effect of diodes-laser silver arsenide-aluminum (Gs-Al-As) 904 nm on healing of experimental wounds. Lasers Surg Med, 7:444–447.

Lopes-Martins R A, Albertini R, Martins P S, Bjordal J M, Faria Neto H C. Spontaneous effects of low-level laser therapy (650 nm) in acute inflammatory mouse pleurisy induced by carrageenan. Photomed Laser Surg. 2005; 23 (4): 377–381.

Lopes-Martins R A, Marcos R L, Leonardo P S, Prianti A C, Muscara M, Aimbire F N, Frigo L, Iversen V V, Bjordal J M. The Effect of Low Level Laser Irradiation (Ga-Al-As - 655nm) On Skeletal Muscle Fatigue induced by Electrical Stimulation in Rats. J Appl Physiol. 2006 Apr 20.

Lubart R, Friedmann H, Faraggt A, and Rochkind 5. (1991): Towards a mechanism of low energy phototherapy. Laser Therapy, 3:11–13.

Lubart R, Friedman H, Grossman N, Cohen N, Breibart H. (1997): The role of reactive oxygen species in photobiostimulation. Trends in Photochemistry and Photobiology, 4:277–283.

Lyons RF, Abergel RP, White RA, Dwyer RM, Castel JC, Uitto J. (1987): Biostimulation of wound healing in vivo by a helium-neon laser. Ann Plast Surg, 18:47–50.

McCaughan JS, Bethel BH, Johnston T, and Janseen W. (1985): Effect of Low Dose Argon Irradiation on Rate of Wound Closure. Lasers in Surgery and Medicine, 5:607–614.

Mendez T M, Pinheiro A L, Pacheco M T, Nascimento P M, Ramalho L M. Dose and wavelength of laser light have influence on the repair of cutaneous wounds. J Clin Laser Med Surg. 2004; 22 (1): 19–25.

Mester E, et al. (1985): The Biomedical Effects of Laser Application. Lasers in surgery and Medicine 5:31–39.

Mester E, Mester AF, Mester A. (1985): The biomedical effects of laser application. Lasers Surg Med, 5:31–39.

Mikhallov VA, Skobelkin O K, Denisov, I N, Frank G A and Voltchenko N N. (1993): Investigations on the influence of low level diode laser irradiation on the growth of experimental tumours. Laser Therapy, 5: 33–38.

Mognato M, Squizzato F, Facchin F, Zaghetto L, Corti L. Cell growth modulation of human cells irradiated in vitro with low-level laser therapy. Photomed Laser Surg. 2004; 22 (6): 523–526.

Mokhtar B, Baxter D, Walsh D, Bell A, Allen J. (1995): Double-blind, placebo-controlled investigation of the effect of combined phototherapy/low intensity laser therapy upon experimental ischaemic pain in humans. Lasers in Surgery and Medicine, 17:74–81.

Monteforte P, Baratto L, Molfetta L, Rovetta G. Low-power laser in osteoarthritis of the cervical spine. Int J Tissue React. 2003; 25 (4):131–136.

Naeser M, Hahn K-A, Lieberman BE, Branco KF. (2002): Carpal Tunnel Syndrome Pain Treated with Low-Level Laser and Microamperes Transcutaneous Electric Nerve Stimulation: A Controlled Study. Archives of Physical Medicine and Rehabilitation, 83:978–988.

Nakaji S, Shiroto C, Yodono M, Umeda T, Liu Q. Retrospective study of adjunctive diode laser therapy for pain attenuation in 662 patients: detailed analysis by questionnaire. Photomed Laser Surg. 2005; 23 (1): 60–65.

Nascimento P M, Pinheiro A L, Salgado M A, Ramalho L M. A preliminary report on the effect of laser therapy on the healing of cutaneous surgical wounds as a consequence of an inversely proportional relationship between wavelength and intensity: histological study in rats. Photomed Laser Surg. 2004; 22 (6):513–518.

Nicola R A, Jorgetti V, Rigau J, Marcos T T. Effect of low-power GaAlAs laser (660 nm) on bone structure and cell activity: an experimental animal study. Lasers in Medical Science 2003; 18 (2): 89–94.

Oren DA, Charney DS, Lavie R, Sinyakov M, Lubart R. (2001): Stimulation of reactive oxygen species production by an antidepressant visible light source. Biol Psychiatry, 49:464–467.

Oron U, Yaakobi T, Oron A, Hayam G, Gepstein L, Wolf T and Ben Haim S. (2001): Attenuation of the formation of scar tissue in rats and dogs post myocardial infarction by low energy laser irradiation. Lasers Surg. Med, 28:204–211.

Oron U, Yaakobi T, Oron A, Mordechovitz D, Shofti R, Hayam G, Dror U, Gepstein L, Wolf T, Haudenschild C and Ben Haim S. (2001): Low energy laser irradiation reduces formation of scar tissue following myocardial infarction in dogs. Circulation, 93:296–301.

Oron U. Photoengineering of tissue repair in skeletal and cardiac muscles. Photomed Laser surg. 2006; 24 (2): 111–120.

Ortutay J, et al. (1998): Psoriatic Arthritis Treatment with low power laser irradiation. A double blind clinical study. Lasermedizin—Laser in Med Surg, 13(3–4):140.

Ozkan N, Altan L, Bingol U et al. Investigation of the supplementary effect of GaAs laser therapy on the rehabilitation of human digital flexor tendons. J Clin Laser Med Surg. 2004; 22 (2):105–110.

Ozdemir F, Birtane M, Kokino S. (2001): The clinical efficacy of low-power laser therapy on pain and function in cervical osteoarthritis. Clin Rheumatol, 20(3):181–4.

Palmgren N, et al. (1991): Low Level Laser Therapy of infected abdominal wounds after surgery. Lasers Surg Med, Suppl 3:11.

Palmgren N, et al. (1989): Low-Power Laser Therapy in Rheumatoid Arthritis. Lasers in Medical Science, 4:193.

Pascu, M.L., Suteanu,S., Ignat, P., Pruna, S., Chitu, A. (1995): Semiconductor lasers in rheumatological treatment, SPIE 246:398–401.

Pinfildi C E, Liebano R E, Hochman B S, Ferreira L M. Helium-neon laser in viability of random skin flap in rats. Lasers Surg Med. 2005; 37 (1): 74–77.

Pogrel MA, Chen JW, Zhang K. (1997): Effects of low-energy gallium-aluminum-arsenide laser irradiation on cultured fibroblasts and keratinocytes. Lasers Surg Med, 20:426–432.

Reddy GK, Stehno-Bittel L, Enwemeka CS. (1998): Laser photostimulation of collagen production in healing rabbit Achilles tendons. Lasers Surg Med, 22:281–287.

Reddy GK, Stehno-Bittel L, Enwemeka CS. (2001): Laser photostimulation accelerates wound healing in diabetic rats. Wound Repair and Regeneration, 9.

Salate A C, Barbosa G, Gaspar P et al. Effect of Ga-Al-As Diode Laser Irradiation on Angiogenesis in Partial Ruptures of Achilles Tendon in Rats. Photomed Laser Surg. 2005; 23 (5): 470–475.

Saunders L. (1995): The efficacy of low-level laser therapy in supraspinatus tendonitis. Clin Rehab, 9:126–134.

Schindl A, et al. (1998): Low intensity laser irradiation improves skin circulation in patients with diabetic microangiopathy. Lasers Surg Med, Suppl. 10:7.

Shimoyama M, Fukida Y, Sjimoyama N, Ijima K, and Mizuguchi T. (1992): Effect of He-Ne laser irradiation on synaptic transmission of the superior cervical sympathetic ganglion in the rat. J Clin Laser Med Surg, 10: 337–342.

Siedentopf C M, , Koppelstaetter F, Haala I A et al. Laser acupuncture induced specific cerebral cortical and subcortical activations in humans. Lasers in Medical Science. 2005; July 1.

Solton P, Young S and Dyson M. (1991): Macrophage responsiveness to light therapy with varying power and energy densities. Laser Therapy, 3:105–111.

Soriano F, Campaña V, Moya M, Gavotto A et al. Photobiomodulation of pain and inflammation on microcrystalline arthropathies: experimental and clinical results. Photomed Laser Surg. 2006; 24 (2): 140–150.

Taguchi T, et al. (1991): Thermographic changes following laser irradiation for pain. Clinical Laser Med Surg, 2(9):143.

Tam G. (1999): Low power laser therapy and analgesic action. J Clin Laser Med Surg, 17(1):29–33.

Thawer HL, and Houghton PE. (1999): Effects of laser irradiation on fetal limb development in vitro. Lasers in Surgery and Medicine, 24(4):285–295.

Tunér J and Hode L. (2002): Laser Therapy—Clinical Practice and Scientific Background. Sweden. Prima Books.

Vasseljen O, et al. (1992): Low level laser versus placebo in the treatment of tennis elbow. Scand J Rehab Med, 24:37. Also in Physiotherapy, 5:329.

Weintraub MI. (1997): Noninvasive laser neurolysis in carpal tunnel syndrome. Muscle & Nerve, 20:1029–1031.

Weiss N, Bibikova A and Oron U. (1994): Expression of desmin in regenerating rat and amphibian skeletal muscles. Lasers Med. Sci, 9:167–171.

Weiss N and Oron U. (1992): Enhancement of muscle regeneration in the rat gastrocnemius muscle by low energy laser irradiation. Anat. Embryol, 186:497–503.

Wong B J, Pandhoh N, Truong M T, Diaz S et al. Identification of chondrocyte proliferation following laser irradiation, thermal injury, and mechanical trauma. Lasers Surg Med. 2005; 37 (1): 89–96.

Xijing W and Yu I C. (1987): Observations on the effect of He-Ne laser Acu point Radiation in Chronic Pelvic Inflammation. Journal of Traditional Chinese Medicine 7(4): 263–265.

Yasuyo M, Toshiyuki I, Toyoshi H, Kazuhiro Y, and Mayumi N. (2000): Effects of Near-Infrared Low Level Laser irradiation on microcirculation. Lasers Surg Med, 27:427–437.

Young S, Bolton P, Dyson M, Harvey W, and Diamantopoulos C. (1989): Macrophage responsiveness to Light Therapy. Lasers in Surgery and Medicine, 9:497–505.

Yu W, Naim JO, Lanzafame RJ. (1997): Effects of photostimulation on wound healing in diabetic mice. Lasers Surg Med, 20:56–63.

Glossary

A

Absorb: To transform radiant energy into a different form, with a resultant rise in temperature.

Absorption: Transformation of radiant energy to a different form of energy by the interaction of matter, depending on temperature and wavelength.

Absorption Coefficient: Factor describing light's ability to be absorbed per unit of path length.

Accessible Emission: The magnitude of accessible laser (or other collateral) radiation of a specific wavelength or emission duration at a particular point as measured by appropriate methods and devices. Also means radiation to which human access is possible in accordance with the definitions of the laser's hazard classification.

Accessible Emission Limit: The maximum accessible emission level limit (AEL) permitted within a particular class. In ANSI Z-136.1, AEL is determined as the product of Accessible Emission times the Maximum Permissible Exposure (MPE) using the area of the limiting aperture (7 mm for visible and near infrared lasers).

Active Medium: Collection of atoms or molecules capable of undergoing stimulated emission at a given wavelength.

Afocal: Literally, "without a focal length"; an optical system with its object and image point at infinity.

Aiming Beam: A laser (or other light source) used as a guide light. Used coaxially with infrared or other invisible light, may also be a reduced level of the actual laser used for surgery or for other applications.

Amplification: The growth of the radiation field in the laser resonator cavity. As the light wave bounces back and forth between the cavity mirrors, it is amplified by stimulated emission on each pass through the active medium.

Amplitude: The maximum value of the electromagnetic wave, measured from the mean to the extreme; simply stated: the height of the wave.

Angle of Incidence (See **Incident Light**)

Anode: An electrical element in laser excitation which attracts electrons from a cathode.

Aperture: An opening through which radiation can pass.

Argon: A gas used as a laser medium. It emits blue/green light primarily at 448 and 515 nm.

Attenuation: The decrease in energy (or power) as a beam passes through an absorbing or scattering medium.

Average Power: The total energy imparted during exposure divided by the exposure duration.

B

Beam: A collection of rays that may be parallel, convergent, or divergent.

Beam Diameter: The distance between diametrically opposed points in the cross section of a circular beam where the intensity is reduced by a factor of $1/e$ (0.368) of the peak level (for safety standards). The value is normally chosen at $1/e2$ (0.135) of the peak level for manufacturing specifications.

Beam Divergence: Angle of beam spread measured in radians or milliradians (1 milliradian = 3.4 minutes-of-arc or approximately 1 mil). For small angles where the cord is approximately equal to the arc, the beam divergence can be closely approximated by the ratio of the cord length (beam diameter) divided by the distance (range) from the laser aperture.

Brightness: The visual sensation of the luminous intensity of a light source. The brightness of a laser beam is most closely associated with the radiometric concept of radiance.

C

Cathode: A negatively charged electrical element providing electrons for an electrical discharge.

CO2 Laser: A widely used laser in which the primary lasing medium is carbon dioxide gas. The output wavelength is 10.6 micrometers in the far infrared spectrum. It can be operated in either CW or pulsed.

Coherence: A term describing light as waves which are in phase in both time and space. Monochromaticity and low divergence are two properties of coherent light.

Collimated Light: Light rays that are parallel. Collimated light is emitted by many lasers. Diverging light may be collimated by a lens or other device.

Collimation: Ability of the laser beam to not spread significantly (low divergence) with distance.

Continuous Mode: The duration of laser exposure is controlled by the user (by foot or hand switch).

Continuous Wave (CW): Constant, steady-state delivery of laser power.

Convergence: The bending of light rays toward each other, as by a positive (convex) lens.

Crystal: A solid with a regular array of atoms. Sapphire (Ruby Laser) and YAG (Nd:YAG laser) are two crystalline materials used as laser sources.

CW: Abbreviation for continuous wave; the continuous-emission mode of a laser as opposed to pulsed operation.

D

Diffuse Reflection: Takes place when different parts of a beam incident on a surface are reflected over a wide range of angles in accordance with Lambert's law. The intensity will fall-off as the inverse of the square of the distance away from the surface and also obey a cosine law of reflection.

Divergence: The increase in the diameter of the laser beam with distance from the exit aperture. The value gives the full angle at the point where the laser radiant exposure or irradiance is $1/e$ or $1/e2$ of the maximum value, depending upon which criteria is used.

Dosimetry: Measurement of the power, energy, irradiance, or radiant exposure of light delivered to tissue.

Duty Cycle: Ratio of total "on" duration to total exposure duration for a repetitively pulsed laser.

E

Electromagnetic Radiation: The propagation of varying electric and magnetic fields through space at the velocity of light.

Electromagnetic Spectrum: The range of frequencies and wavelengths emitted by atomic systems. The total spectrum includes radio waves as well as short cosmic rays.

Electromagnetic Wave: A disturbance which propagates outward from an electric charge that oscillates or is accelerated. Includes radio waves; x-rays; gamma rays; and infra-red, ultraviolet, and visible light.

Electron: Negatively charged particle of an atom.

Emission: Act of giving off radiant energy by an atom or molecule.

Emissivity: The ratio of the radiant energy emitted by any source to that emitted by a blackbody at the same temperature.

Energy: The product of power (watts) and duration (seconds). One watt second = one joule.

Energy (Q): The capacity for doing work. Energy is commonly used to express the output from pulsed lasers and it is generally measured in joules (J). The product of power (watts) and duration (seconds). One watt second = one joule.

Energy Source: High voltage electricity, radio waves, flashes of light, or another laser used to excite the laser medium.

F

Flux: The radiant, or luminous, power of a light beam; the time rate of the flow of radiant energy across a given surface.

Focal Length: Distance between the center of a lens and the point on the optical axis to which parallel rays of light are converged by the laser.

Focal Point: That distance from the focusing lens where the laser beam has the smallest diameter.

Focus: As a noun, the point where rays of light meet which have been reflected by a mirror or refracted by a lens, giving rise to an image of the source. As a verb, to adjust focal length for the clearest image and smallest spot size.

Frequency: The number of light waves passing a fixed point in a given unit of time, or the number of complete vibrations in that period of time.

G

Gas Laser: A type of laser in which the laser action takes place in a gas medium.

Gated Pulse: A discontinuous burst of laser light, made by timing (gating) a continuous wave output—usually in fractions of a second.

Gaussian Curve: Statistical curve showing a peak with normal even distribution on either side. May either be a sharp peak with steep sides, or a blunt peak with shallower sides. Used to show power distribution in a beam. The concept is important in controlling the geometry of the laser impact.

Ground State: Lowest energy level of an atom.

H

Helium-Neon Laser (HeNe): A laser in which the active medium is a mixture of helium and neon. Its wavelength is usually in the visible range. Used widely for alignment, recording, printing, and measuring.

Hertz (Hz): Unit of frequency in the International System of Units (SI), abbreviated Hz; replaces cps for cycles per second.

I

Incident Light: A ray of light that falls on the surface of a lens or any other object. The "angle of incidence" is the angle made by the ray with a perpendicular (normal) to the surface.

Infrared Radiation (IR): Invisible electromagnetic radiation with wavelengths which lie within the range of 0.70 to 1000 micrometers. This region is often broken up into IR-A, IR-B, and IR-C.

Intensity: The magnitude of radiant energy.

Ionizing Radiation: Radiation commonly associated with x-ray or other high energy electromagnetic radiation which will cause DNA damage with no direct, immediate thermal effect. Contrasts with non-ionizing radiation of lasers.

Irradiance (E): Radiant flux (radiant power) per unit area incident upon a given surface. Units: Watts per square centimeter. (Sometimes referred to as power density.)

Irradiation: Exposure to radiant energy, such as heat, x-rays, or light.

J

Joule (J): A unit of energy (1 watt-second) used to describe the rate of energy delivery. It is equal to 1 watt-second or 0.239 calorie.

Joule/cm2: A unit of radiant exposure used in measuring the amount of energy incident upon a unit area.

L

Laser: An acronym for light amplification by stimulated emission of radiation. A laser is a cavity, with mirrors at the ends, filled with material such as crystal, glass, liquid, gas, or dye. A device which produces an intense beam of light with the unique properties of coherence, collimation, and monochromaticity.

Laser Medium (Active Medium): Material used to emit the laser light and for which the laser is named.

Lens: A curved piece of optically transparent material which depending on its shape is used to either converge or diverge light.

Light: The range of electromagnetic radiation frequencies detected by the eye, or the wavelength range from about 400 to 760 nanometers. The term is sometimes used loosely to include radiation beyond visible limits.

M

Micrometer: A unit of length in the International System of Units (SI) equal to one millionth of a meter. Often referred to as a "micron."

Micron: An abbreviated expression for micro meter which is the unit of length equal to 1 millionth of a meter. (See Micrometer.)

Mode: A term used to describe how the power of a laser beam is geometrically distributed across the cross section of the beam. Also used to describe the operating mode of a laser such as continuous or pulsed.

Monochromatic Light: Theoretically, light consisting of just one wavelength. No light is absolutely single frequency since it will have some bandwidth. Lasers provide the narrowest of bandwidths that can be achieved.

N

Nanometer (nm): A unit of length in the International System of Units (SI) equal to one billionth of a meter. Abbreviated nm—a measure of length. One nm equals 10^{-9} meter, and is the usual measure of light wavelengths. Visible light ranges from about 400 nm in the purple to about 760 nm in the deep red.

Nanosecond: One billionth (10^{-9}) of a second. Longer than a picosecond or femtosecond, but shorter than a microsecond. Associated with Q-switched lasers.

Nd:Glass Laser: A solid-state laser of neodymium: glass offering high power in short pulses. A Nd doped glass rod is used as a laser medium to produce 1064 nm light.

Nd:YAG Laser Neodymium:Yttrium Aluminum Garnet: A synthetic crystal used as a laser medium to produce 1064 nm light.

Neodymium (Nd): The rare earth element that is the active element in Nd:YAG lasers and Nd:Glass lasers.

O

Optical Pumping: The excitation of the lasing medium by the application of light rather than electrical discharge.

Optical Radiation: Ultraviolet, visible, and infrared radiation (0.35–1.4 nm) that falls in the region of transmittance of the human eye.

Output Power: The energy per second measured in watts emitted from the laser in the form of coherent light.

P

Phase: Waves are in phase with each other when all the troughs and peaks coincide and are "locked" together. The result is a reinforced wave in increased amplitude (brightness).

Photon: In quantum theory, the elemental unit of light, having both wave and particle behavior. It has motion, but no mass or charge.

Power: The rate of energy delivery expressed in watts (joules per second). Thus: 1 Watt = 1 joule/1 Sec.

Pulse: A discontinuous burst of laser, light or energy, as opposed to a continuous beam. A true pulse achieves higher peak powers than that attainable in a CW output.

Pulse Duration: The "on" time of a pulsed laser. It may be measured in terms of millisecond, microsecond, or nanosecond as defined by half-peak-power points on the leading and trailing edges of the pulse.

Pulse Mode: Operation of a laser when the beam is intermittently on in fractions of a second.

Pulse Repetition Frequency (PRF): The number of pulses produced per second by a laser.

Pulsed Laser: Laser which delivers energy in the form of a single or train of pulses.

Pumped Medium: Energized laser medium.

Pumping: Addition of energy (thermal, electrical, or optical) into the atomic population of the laser medium, necessary to produce a state of population inversion.

R

Radiance Brightness: The radiant power per unit solid angle and per unit area of a radiating surface.

Radiant Energy (Q): Energy in the form of electromagnetic waves, usually expressed in units of joules (watt-seconds).

Radiation: In the context of optics, electromagnetic energy is released; the process of releasing electromagnetic energy.

Reflection: The return of radiant energy (incident light) by a surface, with no change in wavelength.

Refraction: The change of direction of propagation of any wave, such as an electromagnetic wave, when it passes from one medium to another in which the wave velocity is different. The bending of incident rays as they pass from one medium to another (e.g., air to glass).

Ruby: The first laser type; a crystal of sapphire (aluminum oxide) containing trace amounts of chromium oxide.

S

Semiconductor Laser: A type of laser which produces its output from semiconductor materials such as GaAs.

Source: The term "source" means either laser or laser-illuminated reflecting surface, i.e., source of light.

Spot Size: The mathematical measurement of the radius of the laser beam.

Superpulse: Electronic pulsing of the laser driving circuit to produce a pulsed output (250–1000 times per second), with peak powers per pulse higher than the maximum attainable in the continuous wave mode. Average powers of superpulse are always lower than the maximum in continuous wave. Process often used on CO_2 surgical lasers.

T

Threshold: The input level at which lasing begins during excitation of the laser medium.

Transmission: Passage of electromagnetic radiation through a medium.

V

Visible Radiation (light): Electromagnetic radiation which can be detected by the human eye. It is commonly used to describe wavelengths which lie in the range between 400 nm and 700–780 nm. The peak of the human spectral response is about 555 nm.

W

Watt: A unit of power (equivalent to one joule per second) used to express laser power.

Watt/cm2: A unit of irradiance used in measuring the amount of power per area of absorbing surface, or per area of CW laser beam.

Wave: A sinusoidal undulation or vibration; a form of movement by which all radiant electromagnetic energy travels.

Wavelength: The length of the light wave, usually measured from peak to peak, which determines its color. Common units of measurement are the micrometer (micron), and the nanometer.

Y

YAG (Yttrium Aluminum Garnet): A widely used solid-state crystal composed of yttrium and aluminum oxides which is doped with a small amount of the rare-earth neodymium.

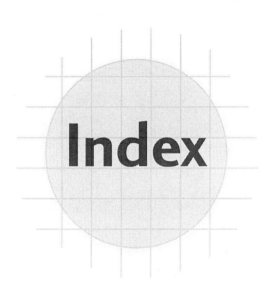

Index